from
SHIP
to
SHORE
&
a whole lot more

MICHELLE CLARKE
with **Helen Kelly**

First published in Great Britain in 2021

Copyright © Michelle Clarke

The moral right of this author has been asserted. All rights reserved.

No part of this publication may be reproduced, stored in a retrieval system, or transmitted, in any form or by any means, without the prior permission in writing of the publisher, nor be otherwise circulated in any form of binding or cover other than that in which it is published and without a similar condition including this condition being imposed on the subsequent purchaser.

Editing, typesetting and publishing by UK Book Publishing
www.ukbookpublishing.com

ISBN: 978-1-914195-27-3

From Ship to Shore & A Whole Lot More

Contents

PART ONE: MICHAEL   1

Chapter 1: Hello World   3
Chapter 2: Junior Years   8
Chapter 3: Family   12
Chapter 4: Grammar School   19

PART TWO: ON BOARD! A MAN'S WORLD   27

Chapter 5: What Have I Done?   29
Chapter 6: Let the Good Times Roll (and Pitch)   43
Chapter 7: A First Time for Everything   50
Chapter 8: Japanese Japes   58
Chapter 9: Scares and Successes   64
Chapter 10: No Sex, Please; We're . . .   72
Chapter 11: I Saw Three Ships   80
Chapter 12: Watch Out!   87
Chapter 13: Love on Land and Sea   97
Chapter 14: XXY   103

PART THREE: CHARTING NEW SEAS — 107

Chapter 15: On the Road — 109
Chapter 16: Hormonal Horrors — 116
Chapter 17: Nude and Rude! — 122
Chapter 18: Blithe Spirit — 130
Chapter 19: Luxury and Loss — 134
Chapter 20: Moving On—In More Ways Than One — 139

PART FOUR: MICHELLE — 147

Chapter 21: To Section or Not to Section? That is the Question — 149
Chapter 22: 'M' for Michelle — 153
Chapter 23: Separation — 158
Chapter 24: All Things Brighton and BUPAful — 164
Chapter 25: Rebellion — 171
Chapter 26: 999 — 178
Chapter 27: A Cheerless Christmas — 182
Chapter 28: SCAM! — 188
Chapter 29: With Friends Like These . . . — 196
Chapter 30: This is Me . . . In a Good Place — 205

Klinefelter Syndrome — 209
Emotionally Unstable Personality Disorder — 211
Acknowledgements and Thanks — 213

Part One

Michael

Chapter 1

Hello World

IF THE CHILDREN'S POEM about the days of the week is to be believed, then Michael, who was born on a Wednesday, would be a child full of woe. And whilst 15 June 1955 was windy and cloudy, it was also a warm day of about 20°C. Children's rhymes and weather reports aside, one might say that Michael was born, to a certain extent, under a cloud, and would experience a good deal, but not a fullness, of woe and chilliness during his life. One might also say that he started life as he meant to go on. Expected at breakfast time, he arrived in time for lunch—his eventual appearance setting the tone for his life: he was late for most of it!

His first memory is from when he was about three years old. He recalls being driven in MC's (a good friend of his family) car with his dad, Jim, and brother, David, to fetch his mum, Edna, and new baby sister, Linda, from the Park Hospital in Wellingborough. Though Linda would grow up to be his closest playmate, all he really remembers about that historical family day was MC's car. It was quite ordinary, in that it was black and had four doors. Unlike other cars, though, it didn't have a boot—just cushions placed on the floor, which Michael and his brother sat upon.

The Park Hospital was a regular feature of Michael's early life, as it was the place where he endured endless trips to take part in lung development exercises. At least twice a week, he recalls, he had to lay on a bed and blow the curtains from about two or three feet away. It was an exercise he had to practise over and over, as well as the closer one of blowing a tissue in the air. Lung exercises in the fifties were clearly unique! It seems likely that nowadays one would just blow into a machine to measure lung capability, but sixty-odd years ago reciting the ditty "I ride my little bicycle, I bought it from the shop, and when I see a big red light, I know I have to stop!" was no doubt considered to be the height of medical science. It worked for Michael anyway, as the walk to the hospital from school with his nan got easier each week.

Though Michael enjoyed his infant school days, he definitely wasn't happy on the day that, like most infants, he soiled himself. He can only think that he couldn't have been fully potty trained, as it only happened to him once. That said, having to return home in borrowed pants and shorts was enough to scar him for life, so he made damn sure he never had to wear the school's spare underwear again!

He was much more fortunate when it came to the dreaded lice checks that anyone from the sixties can recall. The memory of the district nurse setting up in the headmistress, Miss McC's, office, ready to ruffle the heads of hundreds of infants, is one to put fear into most people over 50. Luckily for Michael, his head was always free of lice, so at least he didn't have to endure the humiliation of others knowing he was infested or having some smell recoiling unction rubbed into his skull.

The Victorian school building was handily and happily located opposite a very good sweet shop on Mill Road. Michael remembers going with the penny or twopence that his nan used to give him and buying four-for-a-penny chews—the memory of which brings back the delicious taste to his tongue even now—or a jaw-squeezing Sherbet Dab. Made by Bassett's, the liquorice stick was about the only thing that could stop your face from collapsing in on itself from the sourness of the sherbet. After school Michael loved to pop along to Mr Smith's sweet shop on the corner of Winstanley and Strode Roads. The pennies didn't stay long in Michael's palms before they were quickly swapped for sweets and deposited into Mr Smith's helpful hands. Opposite the sweet emporium was Phillips' the Grocers, who also owned the dairy on Strode Road.

The memory of that dairy is not one that fills Michael with the milk of human kindness, as it was there that one of his greatest fears was instilled in him. Parked in his pram outside—he thinks he can't have been much older than two at the time—a barking dog jumped up at him and frightened him half to death. Though his mum chased the dog away, the fear of what must have felt like a dinosaur's hot mouth trying to devour him has stayed with him so much that 63 years after the event he still doesn't like dogs. The experience didn't put him off other animals though, as he fondly remembers being taken to the zoo on Sheep Street on many occasions by his nan and enjoying it.

Michael had many friends, but the one who had the most unspiritual influence on him was a little girl called EP, whose father was the vicar of the church on Palk Road. Invited to the vicarage by EP, Michael was not expecting her to lock him in the toilet with her when she needed to go. He was so flushed with embarrassment that he didn't know what to do with himself. He could have confided this closet encounter to his favourite teacher, Miss M, but they were young and Michael decided their friendship could prevail over the strange but privy moment.

During 1961 and 1962 Michael used to watch the show *Supercar* which was shown on ITV's children's television. He also used to get the spin-off comic every week and remembers entering a handwriting competition. Why? He doesn't know, as his handwriting was not exactly elegant. Nevertheless, perhaps because there weren't many entries, he won first prize: a trip for his whole family to see a pantomime in London. Unfortunately, Michael caught chicken pox and wasn't able to go, so he was given second prize instead: an LP recording of a story not shown on television.

When he wasn't watching TV, Michael used to enjoy playing with his brother, David, and sister, Linda. When she wasn't watching over them on a Saturday night when their parents went out to The Salon, they would spend a lot of time at their nan's— the wonderfully named Winifred Theodore Tibbetts. Michael really loved his Nan Tibbetts, and in typical noneffusive language describes her as 'a really nice lady'. His enthusiasm for his other nan, meanwhile—Nanna Clarke—requires no effusive outpouring, as he found her to be as cold and exacting as his other nan was warm and understanding. That's not to say that visits to Nanna Clarke were something to be wary of; Michael just had to mind his p's and q's on the few occasions he did visit if he wanted to get a sweet or two from her. Their houses reflected their personalities, so it is no wonder that it was to the warm and welcoming home in Winstanley Road, and not the colder-sounding Elstone Road house, that Michael would go after school.

Though Nan Tibbetts was loving and kind, she would, when the occasion merited it, lay down the law and stop her grandchildren playing if she thought they might get hurt. As she did the time that Michael and David were blowing bubbles, and instead of using the little plastic wand that you dip into the washing-up liquid type mixture, David used his nan's fire poker. Michael can still remember the pain he felt as the poker slammed onto his hand during one particularly feisty bit of bubble bursting. No doubt he felt much better when his nan took him to the baker shop in Mill Road, owned by one of her cousins, where he was handed as many cakes as he could eat.

In the sixties and seventies Wellingborough's population steadily increased due to agreements signed between the Urban District Council and the councils of London, which identified the market town as a popular place to rehouse London's growing Jamaican and Asian communities. Michael is horrified now to recall the time his lovely nan saw a black person crossing Market Street and the derogatory language she used about them. It was, though, a time which lacked understanding of other races and cultures, and were she still living now, Mrs Tibbetts would be much more like her grandson: warm, open, generous and kind to people of all descriptions, regardless of whether they may have filled him with fear or alarm.

Chapter 2

Junior Years

MICHAEL'S FEELINGS OF ALARM and fear reached their height in junior school and came in the shape of MG, his absolute nemesis. Though a very popular boy at school with loads of mates, Michael was, for reasons that are still unfathomable to him today, always picked on by MG.

Bullies tend to be people who have experienced some very difficult times in their own lives and choose to make themselves feel stronger, or just better, by picking on someone else. Unfortunately for Michael, MG decided that he would feel better if Michael gave him his dinner money, and would get it with menaces if not freely given, on an all-too-regular basis. With hunger rumbling his belly, Michael's legs would tremble in unison as the bully returned to continue his nastiness in whichever way, shape or form he decided would work that particular afternoon or morning.

His tormentor always seemed to be around after school too, whenever Michael went to his nan's. Living just around the corner from her in Strode Road, the tyrant took every opportunity to continue to bait his target until, that is, Michael took his good friend, DB, back to Winstanley Road with him. Seeing MG lying in wait, DB lost no time in sticking up for his friend and beat him up. Under sufferance on the floor, DB then encouraged Michael to hurt his bully. An eye for an eye didn't sit well with Michael though, so instead of pouring out his hatred with his fists, he simply emptied his bottle of ink over the supine boy and stood back to watch as the ink leaked into the fabric of his skin through his clothes. No satisfaction was ever greater than at that moment, so the inevitable telling off for ruining another boy's clothes was well worth the worry.

In the third year, Michael had an actual fight which led to much more than a suit of ruined clothes. His friend, DD, and he had an oxymoronic friendly fight. Though amenable in every way, DD was stronger than he looked, so when he threw Michael to the floor, the force knocked out his two front teeth when he landed facedown. It has been a very real reminder to Michael every day since that violence, whether in play or not, doesn't pay. Luckily for him, the dentist, Mr C, who managed to resurrect some semblance of incisors out of the stumps that were left, was an NHS dentist, so at least Michael's parents didn't have to shell out for his new false teeth. Over the years, Michael has had to dig deep though, as his two front teeth have cost him more than a few pounds, especially the nuggets of gold he's worn as crowns. Fortunately, the development of dentistry over the last five decades has reunited Michael with a smile he is fond of.

Michael shared his surname, including the 'e', with his junior school headmaster and found fun in telling people that the top teacher was his dad; though it fell flat when he was dropped off or picked up from school by his real dad in his work's van and someone would say, "Why's he picking you up? I thought your dad was the headmaster." Michael learnt quite quickly that though fun may be had, telling lies doesn't work! He learnt to keep his thoughts to himself and found ways of finding out the facts another way, so when, during one assembly, the headmaster asked the children what words they didn't understand in the hymn they were going to sing, Michael declined to say which one he found odd. Whilst lots of the other kids raised their hands to have unusual terms explained to them, Michael waited until afterwards and asked his friends what his funny word meant. He'd never been to Egypt, let alone heard of it!

The furthest Michael ventured on a daily basis was to school, which being on the other side of town to where he lived was quite a trip. When they were young, mum Edna would travel with all three children on the bus, but as they grew up, older brother David was given the responsibility of delivering his siblings to school and back again. They'd get the bus from just outside their house into town and from there walk the half mile or so to their school. Making the trip in winter was no easy march, and Michael can't imagine being able to trudge through such heavy snow now just to get to school. Mind you, with health and safety so rigorous nowadays, it's unlikely that a child would be expected to make such an irksome journey, and would instead spend his day enjoying that thing that all modern children and teachers long for at least once a season: a snow day!

Though he spent most of his time hanging out with, or avoiding, boys at school, Michael also had several female friends. He particularly remembers a girl called KT, whom he rather fancied. Alas, she didn't feel the same way. They remained friendly though and kept in touch once they'd left school. Michael recalls meeting her in a pub in Great Doddington once. Whilst he'd gone on to get married, she had given her life over to alcohol and drugs. She sadly died about 20 years ago, but Michael still remembers her with fondness. She was a nice person, even if she didn't want to go out with him!

As we grow older and become wiser, the people who have peppered our lives eventually leave, go away and come back, or stay forever. So the day that Michael passed the 11+ matriculation exams was a day of great happiness for him. It meant that he would be going to grammar school and would finally be free of his arch-enemy, MG. It takes a clever person to pass the 11+, so it was not at all surprising that MG's bullying tactics only got him as far as the local secondary modern!

Though a person may be able to physically move on, doing so emotionally is another matter altogether. Research into mental health has found that children who were bullied by other children are at a higher risk of developing mental health difficulties, including depression, anxiety and self-harm. Being bullied by MG has had long-lasting consequences on Michael's mental well-being, which we will explore in later chapters.

Chapter 3

Family

MICHAEL HAD A HAPPY CHILDHOOD with good parents, Edna and Jim, older brother, David, and younger sister, Linda. He was very close to Linda—possibly because she often took the rap for any trouble he got into. All three of them used to play together in the garden with a lad from up the road, but Michael clearly remembers enjoying doing more feminine things just with Linda, like going through the Kays catalogue—his mum was an agent for them, so there were always a few catalogues around—picking out what he wanted or pointing out what he already had.

There was a sandpit just outside their back door that Michael and David used to play in. He remembers once having made some spectacular sandcastles, when all of a sudden moats started gathering around them. The mystery of that particular tide coming in was soon solved when they discovered that a water pipe had burst. Michael was not at all impressed when his sandpit was dug up to repair the damaged pipe.

When he wasn't choosing what he'd like from the catalogue with Linda, or playing in the sandpit with David, the three of them used to pop along to the ABC Minors Club on a Saturday morning at the ABC Cinema on Midland Road. Michael remembers they'd watch cartoons that were quite thrilling and saw *The Lone Ranger* several times. Midland Road was also the destination of the tea room—memorable for its circular window—that Edna would take them to, and where they'd be very sophisticated taking tea, coffee and cakes.

Driving through the town recently, Michael saw his younger self in these buildings; even though the cinema is no longer there and the tea room has been turned into offices, the feelings of the fun they shared all those years ago are just as intense as they were when Michael was a little boy. As he drove past the Castle Theatre, he recalled it was once another kind of auditorium, where cows and pigs were sold under an auctioneer's hammer. Remembering his visits evoked not only intense feelings, but also a very strong sense of smell. On Doddington Road the garage where Michael used to buy Tizer and Jusoda pop is still there, though it no longer sells fuel.

Walking through Wellingborough now is a child's walk through history for Michael. There on Market Street was a ladies' shop called 'Green & Valentine' and on Sheep Street, 'Hordons', Michael's favourite toy shop, where he would browse for hours, choosing which cars he wanted and persuading his parents to buy them. His love of cars may have begun then, or in the back of MC's bootless mobile, and has grown into a keen passion for real motors. And there, too, on Victoria Road is the barbers that he and David used to go to. Haircuts were mandatory for the Clarke brothers: short, back and sides, no doubt, was the barber's commission. Though it was not a pleasant experience for Michael, he valued the care and consideration his stylist took, making him comfortable in the high seat on the barber's chair, so much so that when they became reacquainted years later, his presence in Michael's life was, for him, a very good thing. Michael can still remember Linda's lovely long hair tied in pigtails that reached the small of her back. Whether he desired it or not, he certainly admired it, so his sister's protective manner towards it just made him realise how special it was and how good it looked on her.

Although both his parents worked, Michael remembers that money was tight. Dad, Jim, used to work at the iron foundry in Wellingborough as an electrician before moving to the Central Electric Company. During the war he was a radio operator in the RAF. Michael can remember his dad telling him tales of times he spent in North Africa and Italy and other exotic places, populated by weird and wonderful creatures unheard of in a Northamptonshire market town. He's never forgotten the story of his dad emptying sand out of his boots in the desert to rid the insides of any stowaway scorpions.

Even though Edna was in uniform herself, as a member of the Women's Land Army, Jim must have looked jolly handsome in his RAF uniform as it was—so the family folklore goes—that which attracted Edna to him when they met on a night out on the town. Though her children always came first, she too worked all her life. She had a variety of secretarial roles and worked as a shop assistant at Woollies, where keeping her beady eye on them, she'd allow the children to buy some sweets from the pick 'n' mix counter. Michael's sharpest memory, though, is waiting for her after school whilst she finished her shift at Saxby's. The factory was a great employer who used to organise trips and outings for their workers' families, which Michael remembers with both pride and affection.

As a family they enjoyed many holidays together too, in Torquay and on one occasion at the amusingly named El Cid Hotel in Margate. Michael remembers one particular trip to France with TW, a friend of his parents. They'd borrowed tents from the Scouts, and he shared his with Linda. He wasn't sure Linda thought it was funny when he took the mick out of her for wearing a vest; however, she did—like him—love asking for a bottle of Pschitt at the local shop. Just in case you are wondering, it was a bottle of French pop spelled P-S-C-H-I-T-T!

At home the family loved to spend time together. They had a second-hand cottage suite in the sitting room comprising a two-seater settee and two armchairs. On a winter's night, Jim would make up the coal fire, and with the three kids squeezed on the two-seater, everyone would gather round the warming flames and play cards. Kan-U-Go, a precursor to Scrabble, was a family favourite which Michael remembers gave them hours of fun. And then there was the now-very-collectible card game, Dan Dare, based upon the character in the Eagle comic. The deal was to collect as many tricks as possible, and whoever had the most was declared the winner.

Regardless of who won, the thing that mattered most was that the family were together in harmony around a coal fire that gave as much warmth to them individually as they gave to each other. Jim was extraordinarily proud that his family had a real fire, and though he didn't much like emptying the ashes of a morning, getting it started on an evening and keeping the embers stoked and his family warm was all that mattered. He must have been horrified the day a group of boys playing by the tree-lined brook on Doddington Road, not far from their house in Valley Road, set fire to one of the trees. The fire brigade were called, and no doubt the police had something to say about it. Setting majestic flora aflame must be one of the most heinous acts of environmental vandalism to witness; finding out that your younger son was not part of the gang must have been some small consolation.

Michael can still, in his mind's eye, see his dad down on the floor playing with David's ninth birthday present with him. It was a set of Bayko building equipment, and they had great fun making things together. It's a memory Michael treasures, as, as dads and sons sometimes do, Jim and David grew apart as adults. He also recalls that his dad had a pretty nifty NSU Prinz moped which he used to go to work on. For a bit of fun, he'd take the boys for a spin around the block on it. Standing on the footplates as he whizzed along was exhilarating.

Pushbikes, too, were a set of wheels Michael was secure on, even if the bike in question was too big for him. Long before he owned his own bike, he used to borrow his mum's old one, which his Nan Tibbetts kept in her junk-filled front room. Despite being a ladies' racing bike, Michael used to peddle it up and down the street like he was the king of the mountain, though whether he wore a polka-dot shirt then, or waited until later, remains to be seen.

From a single street, to going much further afield to Chelveston and other faraway places with his brother David, and when Linda was given her new bike after passing the 11+, he also went out and about with her. On one occasion they cycled to Wicksteed Park in Kettering and had some fun on the free facilities. With the day turning mild, Michael didn't need his cycling gloves, so he thought he would put them in his sister's saddlebag. Linda was not having that, and an argument ensued. It wasn't just the bike gloves that were off! Not wanting to fight with his sister, Michael cycled off and left her. Once he'd calmed down, he found her again and the sibling rivalry was settled.

When he wasn't riding around, he could be found out and about with the Cubs or Scouts. As a member of the St Andrew's troop in Wellingborough, he can remember having great fun, and though he can't remember their names, he can clearly picture both his Akela and Bagheera. He progressed to being a patrol leader and was proud to be able to lead his own team. It's a little surprising that such a responsible sounding lad would then get into trouble with the law when he was caught carving his initials into a tree not far from where he lived. Well-known local bobby, BW, put the frighteners on him when he caught him red-handed, so it was a big relief for Michael to find that he hadn't actually been reported when he got home.

Home was a safe haven for Michael, and a place that his wider family and friends loved to pop in. Uncle Eddie, his dad's twin, and Auntie Jean were frequent guests, as was his father's younger brother, Uncle Jeffrey. Of course, visits were reciprocated, though not always relished, especially when it involved a five-mile walk from Wellingborough to Rushden to see hairdresser Auntie Jean in her shop. Welcome refreshments and knowing that their dad was going to pick them up in his car made the walk worthwhile though. Closer to home the boys would often drop in on their Great Auntie Nell, who lived in the Alms Houses on Doddington Road. Her one-bedroom flat, with its roaring open fire, was a very cosy place to go, even if it was located opposite the cemetery.

AA, the Co-op delivery-van man, though not family or friend, was always welcome when he did his rounds on a Thursday evening. Edna would take the children out and let them choose some chocolate each—a Mars bar perhaps or a Kit Kat. Lots of luxuries were delivered direct to the door in the seventies, which Michael and his siblings loved. None more so than the fizzy pop that was delivered by Cooks Drinks, though of course being connoisseurs of the fashionable liquid, it was the real deal Corona which they chose as opposed to the own brand. Whilst not a luxury, having your milk delivered by a horse-drawn float nowadays would certainly feel like it. Fifty years ago, horse-drawn carriages were dying out, so being visited upon by a beautiful high-hands beast may still have been a treat. Sadly, not for Michael, who found the horse quite scary and is wary around them even now.

Then there was the bread man who brought Edna her single-tin loaf once a week, and the coalman who, black as night, would drop their ton of coal into the coalhouse outside the back door. And through that door, EC—no connection except as their next door neighbour—and her trusty hound, Rusty, often popped in to play. From across the road another friend, RB, would also wander over to spend happy hours with Michael and his siblings.

We are lucky in life if we are able to reach adulthood without the spectre of death's shadow dropping in on us. Sadly, the grim reaper didn't spare Michael an early visit, but came twice during his young life: on the occasion he stole RB away, and then again when he took his still-young Auntie Jean from those she loved.

At the time of RB's demise, Michael was preparing for or taking his 11+. When he passed he was rewarded for his efforts by his parents—as were his siblings when they, too, passed—with a new bike. His reward, though, was actually twofold, as passing the test meant he could go to Wellingborough Grammar School for Boys and thus was able to finally speed away from his relentless bully, MG, and start afresh at his next school.

Chapter 4

Grammar School

THOUGH IT WAS A NEW START, Michael's feelings towards school didn't change much: he still hated it and was late every day of every year. This was largely because they had assemblies every morning, which to his mind were a complete waste of time, so he stayed in bed for an extra 20 minutes instead. You can imagine how many detentions he clocked up when eventually the headmaster would say, "Not you again. Go away, Clarke!"

He began at the school in September 1966 and finished in March 1972. Though he started off well in the highest class, 1A, he was deemed not bright enough to continue, so at the end of the first term was transferred to 1B. Though he worked hard, at the end of the second term, he was dropped again into 1 Beta, or what Michael self-deprecatingly calls 'the lowest grade for dummies like me'. Though he didn't know it at the time, Klinefelter's, which he was diagnosed with much later in life, causes slow academic development. This clearly had an impact on Michael throughout his school days.

He was good at maths, which he enjoyed, and not bad at English; though, again in that self-scornful way of his, he thinks he was rubbish at lots of other things. Physics, he got on well with, but history was an anathema. He was so disinterested in the past that he only managed to gain nine per cent in his mock O-level exam.

Michael wasn't a great fan of PE, but it was a drastic step to get out of it by developing an abscess on his left upper arm in the first year. He ended up going to Northampton General Hospital to have the offending carbuncle drained under general anaesthetic. Rather than being afraid, he found it all quite exciting. Going to the hospital with his mum and dad in the work's van to do more than blow a pair of curtains was exciting enough, but having an operation was a great adventure. Following the procedure, as his dad had gone back to work, he and his mum were taken home in an ambulance. It might have been an excellent adventure, but puking the effects of the anaesthetic into a kidney dish in the back of the ambulance was a quest too far!

A few days later he had to go to the doctors on the High Street to have the abscess checked. When the doctor undid the dressings, he pulled loads of bandage out of the hole in his arm, just like a conjuror pulling hankies out of a hat. The magic hadn't quite worn off as much as he thought. How could all of that be coming out of his arm? he wondered. He couldn't believe his eyes, and nearly passed out. The scar, a constant reminder of his first operation, is also a badge of honour—surely a winner in the 'show me your best scar' competition!

Being a grammar school, there were many options for a varied curriculum. In his first year he learnt to play chess in the weekly class taught by Mr N. A few years later he joined the photographic society and, using the school projector which he set up in a large classroom, took it upon himself to show films during the lunch hour. Michael's entrepreneurial skills are explored further in Part 3, and it might be fair to say that his talent for setting up successful projects started at school. Entrance to the lunchtime screenings were 50 pence per person, and for that the audience would be able to watch a variety of films, both educational and non. One of the most successful films Michael showed was a factual presentation called *Policeman* all about the work of the police force, which seemed to appeal to both the clever grammar school boys and their teachers.

Michael's teachers were, even though they would send him on litter-picking duty for being late, in many ways full of praise him. His second year maths teacher nominated him for the end-of-year prize for being top of his class, for which Michael received a book of his choice. It was presented and signed by David Frost—one of the school's famous 'old boys'. In the third year his English teacher, and subsequently fourth-form master, Mr W, was always pleased to share his love of toy cars and lorries with his student, often photographing Michael's Corgi and Dinky toy collections, which he'd bring in to show him, and displaying them on the classroom wall. Sadly, Mr W passed away when Michael was in the fifth year, but he's never forgotten their mutual interest in cars and will always remember him driving his antique Berkeley Three-Wheeler.

It was often their cars which drew Michael to a particular member of staff, and though he recalls the school secretary as a rather large and officious lady who ran his sister's Brownie group, he remembers her little blue Austin A35 more fondly. Though it wasn't his car that sticks in Michael's mind, it was travel that endeared his music teacher, Mr C, to him. As a member of the school choir, he was chosen to sing for the county in a travelling choral group made up of students from other schools. Michael was just one of two boys from the grammar school to sing with the choir at various churches within the county, which they travelled to by coach.

In the seventies schools were much more relaxed than they are now. Safeguarding was not high on the agenda, and teachers were largely allowed to drive students in their cars without having to worry about false allegations being made against them or ensuring that a chaperone was present. There was more trust in the profession, and teachers and their families, like the fictional good old 'Mr Chips', could be much more welcoming towards their students outside of school. TG and his wife, K, lived not far from Michael and were on his weekly round when he delivered lottery tickets for Cancer Research. Michael got on very well with the Gs, who kept in touch with him by letter long after he'd stopped travelling the world on board ship.

School wasn't all work and no play. Back together with his junior school friend, DB, and finding new mates in BH, RA and AF, he spent quite a lot of time with them both in and out of school. Mostly, things went really well, except on the occasion when he went home with AF, who lived near him. Stopping at AF's, they met up with a boy from another school and went off to his house to hang out—except that the old 'two's company, three's a crowd' adage got in the way, and when the other two wouldn't let Michael join in, he gently threw a stone at the boy's front window. He only threw it underarm with very little force: his intention being to just get their attention. Well! He certainly did that all right—when the stone went right through the window and into the lounge. Michael was in shock!

Not wanting to stay and admit what his little jealous outburst had done, he jumped on his bike and rode home as fast as he could. He didn't dare tell his parents and hoped that his 'crime' would go unnoticed. He should have remembered that telling lies, or in this case withholding the truth, doesn't pay, as at about 7 pm that evening the other boy's parents came to his house and asked his dad to pay for the damage. Michael remembers the words that issued forth under his breath: "Oh shit!" Fortunately, though his dad was not best pleased with him, he didn't give him a good hiding. The 17 shillings and sixpence it cost for the replacement window was something they could ill afford, but more lives are lost at sea than they ever are from breaking a window in a fit of jealous pique. Michael never saw the other boy again, but like his family, his friend AF stayed loyal to him.

Loyalty to your cycling buddy, especially when doing trips of 120 miles or more, makes clocking up the miles on your bike much more fun and enjoyable. Michael remembers two occasions when he and his good friend, DB, rode to the seaside for a bit of sun, sea and sand. Staying overnight in their tent, along with another friend, GP, it took them two days to reach the coast, where they pitched for a week and explored Cromer before cycling back. The return journey was not quite as straightforward as the ride forth. When GP sped off, Michael and DB were left to look after themselves. Getting as far as Eye, near Peterborough, they decided to set up camp. Realising that they didn't have the poles for their tent—either GP had them or they'd got lost en route—caused a major problem. Stopping at a local garage to get some help, they soon found themselves in the back of a police van being whisked off to the local station.

Responding to a call from the garage owner about two 15-year-old lads on the road without their poles, the police kindly took them off to Peterborough, where they spent the night in the cells. They had a cell each and were told that unless somebody whose behaviour was not as innocent as theirs was picked up, the cell doors would remain open. Clearly, that night there were some naughty people picked up in Peterborough, as when the boys woke their doors were locked. The kind bobbies, realising they were awake, served them a breakfast of tea and toast before waving them off to Wellingborough on their bikes. Being far more experienced, their second trip to Clacton went smoothly, and though they had a good time in the Essex town, their journey back required no police intervention.

The same can't now be said for other situations Michael was involved in. He had, since he was a small boy, been having his hair cut by the same barber on Victoria Road. Michael liked him and felt safe in his company, though his intentions in boys lay in more than just cutting their hair. On occasions he would cycle to his house after school, where his attentions were more than just friendly. Though Michael knew deep down that it was wrong, he felt good about it, so he never told his parents or friends. As he grew older and he learnt that his barber had close liaisons with other teenage boys, his interest in him waned and he switched to a men's hairdresser in Sheep Street.

All teenagers experience tumultuous hormonal changes, and finding out what they like, especially when it comes to sex, is normal. When he was 16 Michael became attracted to a chap, BP, he met through the Scouts. Though three years older than Michael and a leader of another Scout pack, they got on extremely well. He had a motorbike and would often pick Michael up from school on it. They would go to the Queen's Head pub in Oxford Street, where Michael tasted his first pint of beer—even though at 17 he was underage, the landlord turned a blind eye. Though he has been married to IB for 30 years, BP remains Michael's closest and dearest friend today.

Though Michael managed to blag his way out of assemblies and got away with detentions, his real punishment caught up with him later when he only managed to pass two O-levels in English and Maths—the other factor being that he couldn't be bothered to revise. He'd flicked through the *School Leaver*, a small magazine designed to entice students into all sorts of different careers. Over half of the adverts were from shipping companies looking for deck/navigation or engineering cadets. Not fancying engineering, he was quite taken with the idea of being a navigation officer, so he decided he wanted to join the Merchant Navy.

Being averse to companies that owned oil tankers or passenger ships—he didn't like the idea of transporting oil or looking after the rich and famous—he applied to Sir William Reardon Smith & Sons Ltd, a small non-hazardous goods shipping company based in Cardiff. His application in 1971 was well received, and he was called for an interview. As he'd never travelled far from home on his own, and the long train journey included a change in London, mum Edna went with him. They stayed in a hotel overlooking Cardiff Castle, then the next morning went to Devonshire House in Greyfriars Road where Michael was introduced to the company training officer, GB, and the interrogation began. When asked the inevitable, future-probing, tricky interview question, "Where do you expect to be in three years' time?" Michael quickly quipped, "Third officer!"—and they agreed to take him on.

His academic past suddenly caught up with him when he realised he would need four O-levels to join. As pride comes before a fall, he returned to school and asked to redo the fifth year, which the headmaster, HW, agreed to. This time he knuckled down to his studies and was rewarded with a further two passes in geography and physics. His compass was set!

When he was 15 Michael got a Saturday job in the hardware department at the Co-op in Wellingborough. As selling household and small kitchen items didn't really float his boat, he soon switched to the electrical department, where he enthused over washing machines and hoovers, toasters and hi-fi systems to his customers. Enjoying his role and having a good rapport with his colleagues, he took on a full-time position during the summer before starting his induction training in September.

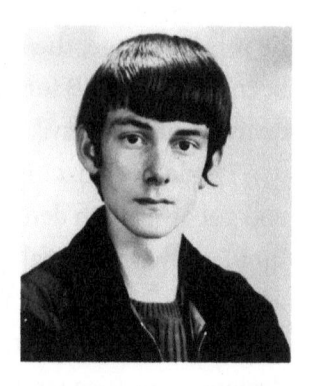

Me at about 15 years old

Keen to learn to drive, he began taking double lessons on his 17th birthday and passed his test first time six weeks later. Clearly happy with him, his manager, DC, allowed him to drive the delivery van, which Michael felt was a great achievement. Mr C was obviously a man who understood the needs of young people, so Michael was pleased to hear that he later went on to become a lecturer at Wellingborough College. When he finally left to take up his commission, the staff in the electrical department gave Michael a cassette radio to take with him. It was probably one of the best and most companionable things he took aboard.

Part Two

On Board!
A Man's World

Chapter 5

What Have I Done?

BEFORE HE WAS ALLOWED to attend his induction course, Michael had to keep an appointment at the Mercantile Marine Office in London, where he was to sit a very rigorous eye test. If he wasn't able to see pinprick lights and recognise colours, all bets would be off. Having never travelled on a long journey alone, his mum accompanied him, so when he did pass the test she was there to congratulate him. The final requirement Michael needed to fulfil was to become a fully paid-up member of The Merchant Navy And Airline Officers Association (MNAOA)—the union of the Merchant Navy which would ensure that he would always be supported whilst at sea.

Finally the day arrived for Michael to leave home. With all his equipment packed in an oversized suitcase, he set off in full winter uniform on Thursday 7 September 1972. For the first time in his life he was all alone on a long journey, and even though he was embarking on a new, exciting adventure, he couldn't stop the tears from falling as he left his mum, dad and sister on the train station platform. He told himself, "It's only for two weeks, and then I'll be back." But nevertheless he felt like his heart was being ripped out of his chest; it was so hard to accept.

When he arrived at the Plymouth School of Maritime Studies, he was designated a bed in a dormitory of six in the college halls of residence. Michael liked to stay in bed of a morning, so one can only imagine what his first wake-up call must have been like. The commander in charge of the cadets—an ex-Royal Navy petty officer—clearly had experience in getting new cadets out of their bunks. At 7 am sharp a ship's bell would ring over the tannoy, followed by the message, "Hands off cocks, and onto socks!" Clearly a message tailored for boys, but since there were also female cadets amongst the 11 floors of bedrooms, one can only imagine what the girls must have thought. Discriminatory? Or perhaps the commander was covering all bases!

In Plymouth the cadets were taught basic seamanship, which included tying knots, splicing rope, nautical terminology and rowing! They used to go out from the college's marine base in Cattedown in open whalers to learn how to row in unison and how to 'ship oars'. Rowing was tough because the heavy whalers needed a lot of effort to make them move through the water, but Michael rose to the challenge and thoroughly enjoyed it. Though he couldn't swim, being so close to the water didn't frighten him.

Two weeks soon passed, and before he knew it Michael was back on the train home—this time not a frightened 'kid' venturing out into the wide world alone, but a seasoned mariner. Or so he thought. With three weeks' paid leave before he had to join his first ship, he enjoyed being back in the bosom of his family, spending his handsomely weekly wage of £18 on them.

WHAT HAVE I DONE?

Michael's flights, in the first week of October, to Johannesburg and then Durban to join his first ship, the *MV Welsh City*, were a rude introduction to the kind of unit he was joining. Being young and naïve, he hadn't realised that he didn't have to wear full uniform on the plane, so the hours of being laughed at by his fellow officers turned into an awfully long six months at sea.

Though the first cargo was sweet, the week loading the molasses was not. Being of a feminine stature, Michael was not as outwardly manly as his shipmates and not as spritely. The name-calling began almost immediately: 'Splitpin' because he was tall and skinny, and 'Flash' because he was slower than everyone else. Starting a new career in a new country, with a host of intimidating

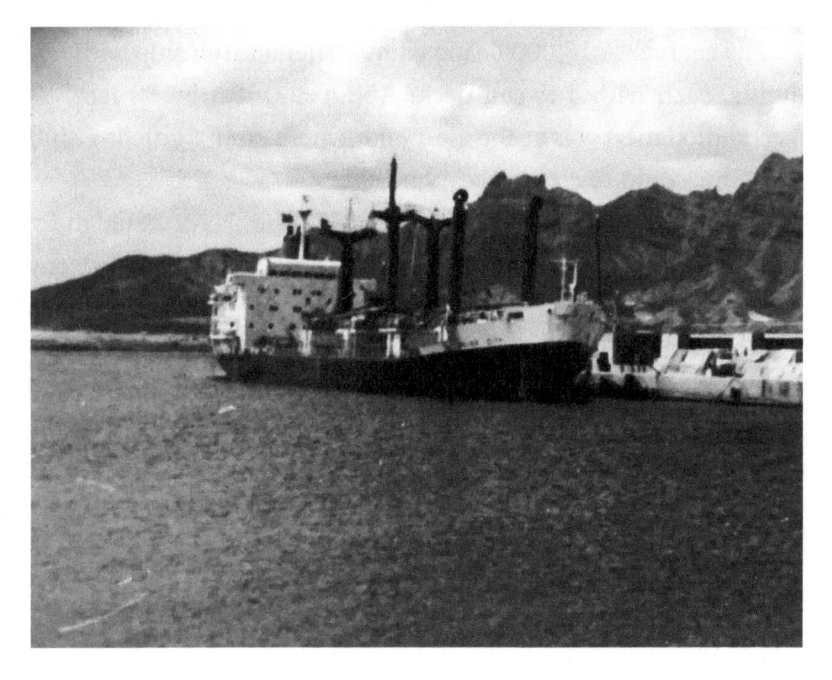

My first ship - MV Welsh City

sailors, soon took its toll. When asked to use a rope ladder to climb down from the poop deck to water level to read the draft, Michael froze on the ladder about six feet down from the ship and had to be coaxed back up. During that first week he wrote home to say how unhappy he was and to ask if his parents could buy him out of the Merchant Navy. It was six weeks before they received his letter.

His cabin, a ten-foot by eight-foot haven, contained a single bunk with drawers under, a single wardrobe, a 'day bed', a sink and a window not a porthole. The toilets and showers were opposite and shared with the other two cadets, one of whom, CS, was also a first-timer. The ship's complement consisted of 16 officers altogether and 30 Indian crew members. The captain, a man who should have been totally looking after his newbie cadets, was, it turned out, a man named for his nature: Captain 'Piggy' B. His charge? A 16,000 deadweight[1] general cargo ship with five holds, each with a tween deck. About 500 feet by 80 feet, its accommodation was at the after end, where after a grueling shift the crew could rest their weary heads.

You would think that being in the Merchant Navy would mean that a person would need to be a strong swimmer with a strong stomach. You'd be wrong. Michael could neither swim nor keep the contents of his stomach down. As the *Welsh City* left Durban and entered the Indian Ocean, a heavy swell made the ship roll and pitch. Michael instantly got seasick. The chief officer took him up to the foc's'le in the hope that the extreme movements of the bow would cure his sickness, but it didn't—he got worse. Thinking he still had the right antidote to his cadet's severe sickness, he took

---

1 Deadweight is the amount of cargo, in tonnes, that the ship can carry.

him higher still, up to the monkey island, where the rolling motion of the ship was accentuated. It made Michael even worse. He finally conceded and allowed Michael to go to his cabin to sleep it off. It took three days before he was able to stand without throwing up. The sickly sweetness of the ship's cargo didn't help; its smell is something that still leaves Michael feeling queasy.

Sailing from Durban to Tokyo in Japan, the ship crosses the equator. Known as 'crossing the line', this course turns into a rite of passage for all first time sailors at the hands of the old timers. For Michael, already the brunt of the ship's sick humour, it was an unpleasant ordeal. Both he and CS were set upon, tied to a makeshift table over some bollards on the poop deck, hosed down with a seawater fire hose then doused in foul-smelling gunk from head to toe. It was made up of fish oil, tar, red lead paint, engine oil and anything else that was hard to remove. Michael was coated all over with this gunk; so much, that he had to throw away his boiler suit. Using a whole tub of Swarfega and nearly two bars of soap, it took him over two hours in the shower to get clean again. Everyone else but Michael thought it was funny! By comparison CS got off lightly. It only took him 20 minutes in the shower to get clean. Had he been more macho or butch, Michael feels he, too, might have got off more lightly. As it was, he was lucky that the captain finally took his responsibilities seriously when he stopped his officers from shaving half of Michael's hair off. A small blessing was that having 'crossed the line' once, Michael was then exempt from undergoing such humiliation every time he crossed the equator.

The persecution he felt came in the form of being picked on, bullied and verbally abused. Everyone was at liberty to have a go, even the captain. However, there were times when Michael found things more bearable: during evening meals and at breakfast time. With allocated places at tables bolted to the deck, in a 'proper' dining room, the atmosphere was calm. Served by Indian stewards, who catered for their every need, officers ate four-course breakfasts off tables decked with crisp white linen cloths and meticulously laid out cutlery. Compared to lunch, served in the 'duty mess', the evening ambience was even more exalted. Sailors were expected cleaned and dressed in the uniform dictated by the climate—tropical whites when it was hot; dress uniform when it was cold—to sit down to their five-course meal, consisting of fruit juice, soup with bread and butter, a choice of main course, dessert and a tea or coffee, at 5.30 pm each day. Should any officer still feel hungry, then sandwiches were always available later in the evening. For any member of the crew at sea over Christmas, then Christmas Day lunch was an even more extravagant affair. A full six-course lunch, with drinks in the captain's cabin. Though not a religious affair, as religion and politics are topics frowned upon on board ship, it was nearly always a jolly event.

The ship had an officer's bar, which was not unlike a pub but on a much smaller scale. Unlike ordinary ales, lager does not spoil with a ship's movements, so ships tend to carry copious amounts. The bar also carries optics of the most common spirits plus various soft drinks. The crew would pay and record what they had from the bar by putting a signed form in the cash box once they were finished. Unlike other officers, Michael didn't drink much alcohol, which gave his shipmates just another reason to poke fun at him. On an evening, between the hours of eight and 12, there could be six to eight officers downing liberal amounts of lager—sometimes as many as a hundred cans between them—and Michael would be the only one on soft drinks. Nowadays there

WHAT HAVE I DONE?

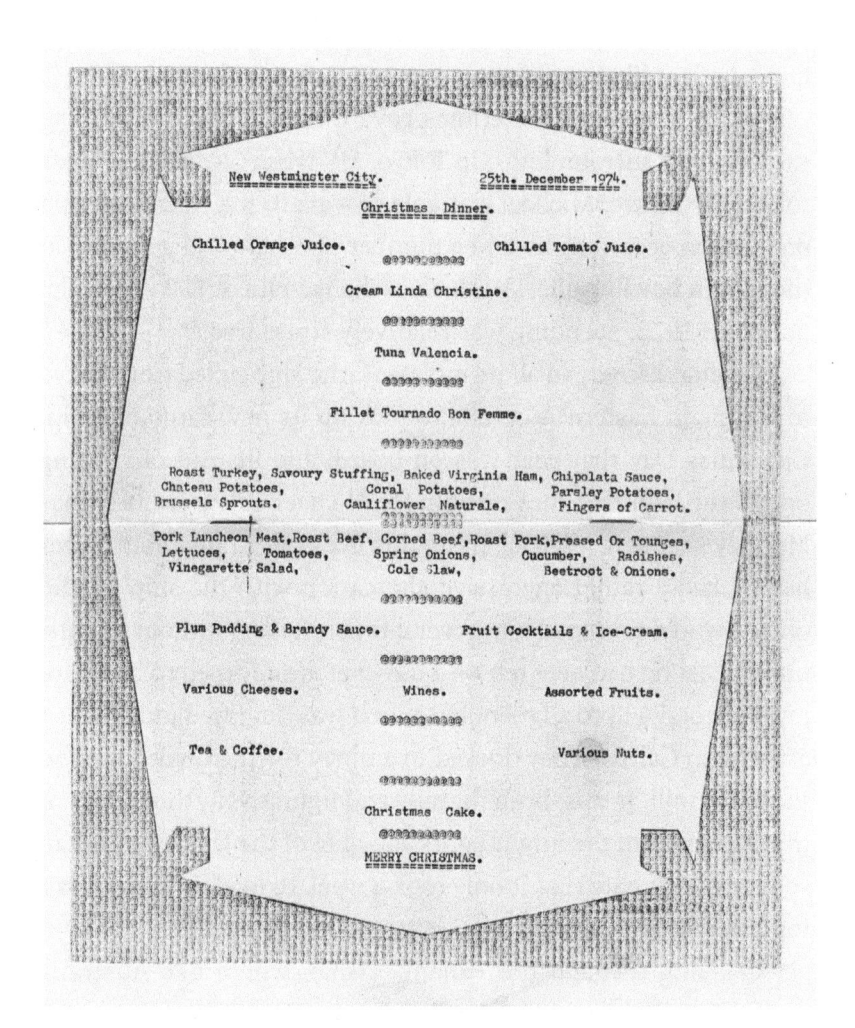

```
New Westminster City.                    25th. December 1974.
                    Christmas Dinner.

     Chilled Orange Juice.              Chilled Tomato Juice.

                    Cream Linda Christine.

                         Tuna Valencia.

                    Fillet Tournado Bon Femme.

   Roast Turkey, Savoury Stuffing, Baked Virginia Ham, Chipolata Sauce,
   Chateau Potatoes,        Coral Potatoes,       Parsley Potatoes,
   Brussels Sprouts.        Cauliflower Naturale,    Fingers of Carrot.

   Pork Luncheon Meat, Roast Beef, Corned Beef, Roast Pork, Pressed Ox Tounges,
   Lettuces,   Tomatoes,     Spring Onions,    Cucumber,   Radishes,
   Vinegarette Salad,        Cole Slaw,        Beetroot & Onions.

     Plum Pudding & Brandy Sauce.     Fruit Cocktails & Ice-Cream.

        Various Cheeses.            Wines.           Assorted Fruits.

        Tea & Coffee.                                Various Nuts.

                         Christmas Cake.

                         MERRY CHRISTMAS.
```

Typical Christmas Menu

are strict rules on how much alcohol a sailor is allowed to imbibe in any one 24 hour period, so the binge drinking that often led to unruly and bullying behaviour towards Michael would, one would hope, be less likely to happen.

Unloading cargo sometimes gave the crew opportunities to explore their surroundings. In Tokyo, *MV Welsh City* berthed close to the city centre. Michael was able to walk to the Ginza,[2] and on one or two occasions he and a number of others had good fun at the tenpin bowling alley. With an exchange rate of 750 yen to the pound in 1972, spending was relatively stress free.

Having discharged all its molasses, the ship sailed from Tokyo to Cairns in Eastern Australia to pick up its new cargo of grain. Christmas Day that year was on board, and instead of it being one of the happier times on ship for Michael, it was a Christmas Monday that saw Michael crying his eyes out in his cabin. After having had a rather aggressive altercation with the ship's radio officer, who'd thumped him several times, it was, without fail, the unhappiest he had ever felt on a day that is supposed to be full of joy and good will to all men. His mood was not lifted much when arriving in Cairns. They docked in a dingy town crowded around the grain mill. It was, both literally and figuratively, thousands of miles away from the bright lights and glitz of the Japanese capital, so it was fortunate that it only took a week to load up and set sail for Canada.

Cruising through the Panama Canal, where like Australia the temperatures remained a deliciously hot 30°C, coming into St John's in New Brunswick was a shock to the system. The

---

2 Japanese for shops.

temperatures had not only dropped, but plummeted to minus 25°C. It was so cold that the ship's heating system froze up and there was no heating in the cabins for several days. The ship's engine room, with all the equipment and things generating local heat, even dropped to being very cold, and the engineers had to wear duffle coats whilst they worked, just to keep warm.

On deck it was even ghastlier. Though the air temperature was minus 25°C, the wind chill and the falling snow made it feel significantly colder. For the Indian Crew it was not just terrible, but life threatening. Not used to such extreme temperatures, they were only allowed out for an hour at a time for their own safety. At the start of each working day ice had to be chipped off the cargo hatches just to get access to the grain. With the daily ice thaw almost a ritual, it was a bitterly slow way to unload, with the month in Canada feeling more like an eternity.

On the one day it didn't snow and the sun shone, the midday temperature crept up to zero centigrade. It was so comparatively warm that the officers all donned their shorts and played football on the quayside. Michael may have wished for such a tropical temperature the night he ventured into a nearby town to meet a girl. Leaving the bar to find all the buses had stopped running, and with no money to get a taxi back to his ship, he walked five miles through the snow and sub-zero temperatures just to get back. Looking back on that now, he wishes he were still so fit!

St John's is famous for having a reversing waterfall, and although Michael didn't go to see it, others did, and their description of this natural wonder left Michael feeling as though he had witnessed it himself. Depending on the time of day, and because of the unique tides in that region, the water flows in one direction and then the other multiple times a day. Despite this wonderful phenomenon, Michael was happy to leave the freezing conditions behind. Sailing empty, they set off on the return voyage to South Africa. Stopping off at the Cape Verde Islands to take on fuel, they experienced another extreme shock to the system. In the 10 days it took to reach the Cape Verdes the temperature rocketed from minus 25°C to plus 30°C.

Michael remembers the Cape Verdes as being a range of beautiful mountains sprouting out from the sea in the middle of nowhere. Unfortunately, he wasn't able to go ashore, as the six to eight hours it took to fill the fuel tanks was too short. Eventually, the ship arrived in Durban once more, took on a load of grain bound for India and sailed to Calcutta up the River Hooghli. A side stream of the Ganges, Michael recalls seeing a dead body floating past the ship as they made their way along the river towards Calcutta. It was perhaps a metaphor for how he was feeling at the end of his first trip.

After a four-hour handover to the replacement complement of officers waiting for them, Michael, his fellow crewmembers and all their luggage were collected by Ambassador Taxis and taken to the Hotel Oberoi Grand for a night's rest before flying back to London the next day. Michael remembers going to his room and falling asleep almost immediately. He didn't wake up for more than 12 hours, he was so exhausted. His flight home passed in a daze, but when he was met by his mum and family friend, BA, who had driven her to the airport to collect him, he perked up considerably. It didn't last long. On the way home he told them how much he hated being in the navy and left them in no doubt whatsoever that he wasn't going back; not just because of the bullying he had experienced, but because every time he left port he felt so tremendously seasick. His mother kept her own counsel in the hope that, after six weeks leave on full pay, he would have a change of heart.

One hundred pounds in 1973 was a lot of money, and the sum Michael had left after six months at sea. By contrast, had he have been in the Royal Navy, he would have had just 10 days' leave. Of course, whilst the Royal Navy is the navy that everyone thinks of, the Merchant Navy plays a big part in the movement of cargoes and people around the world. To compare the two is easy: the Royal Navy ships spend around eight months each year in refit and four months on active duty, whereas the Merchant Navy ships spend two weeks in dry dock, or less, and eleven and a half months on active duty. There is also a big pay difference, with the Merchant Navy consistently paying more per person at all officer ranks. The officer uniforms are remarkably similar, except that where the Royal Navy has roundels on the badge of rank, the Merchant Navy has diamonds.

Six weeks' paid leave may sound like heaven to some, but it was a very lonely time for Michael, as his friends on Civvy Street were all out at work during the day. However, he found ways to keep himself amused during the daytime and had fun socialising in the evenings.

His good friend, BP, took a week off work and together they went camping in the local countryside near Hardwick, just outside Wellingborough. The land was owned by a farmer friend of BP's, which was handy as they were able to get fresh milk from the cow every day. In their two tents, once again borrowed from the Scouts, they were happy and comfortable.

Though he'd met up with a girl in New Brunswick, Michael was sexually attracted to males too. His feelings towards BP grew, and though he wanted to get physical with him, he knew it wouldn't happen as BP had found a girlfriend who visited him most evenings, leaving Michael to imagine what they were up to!

Being a keen hunter, BP took his shotgun along and they were able to dine on pigeon breast cooked over the campfire. On one day Michael's father visited them and decided that he, too, would have a go at shooting pigeons. He didn't quite expect the recoil the gun had, which sent him backwards, though it served as a valuable lesson to Michael, who knew that he'd have been knocked off his feet if he'd had a go.

All through his leave, Michael kept telling his parents how much he hated life on board ship, reiterating how he didn't want to go back. It would have cost his parents £100, a sizeable sum, to buy him out, and that on top of money they had spent on his uniform and other kit was money they just couldn't afford. After talking things through, helping Michael to see that he had just had a bad experience, they finally convinced him to set sail again. Michael agreed on the proviso that if he still felt the same after the next trip, they would indeed buy him out.

In the Reardon Smith Line, all the company-owned ships were called something 'City'. In collaboration with the Mexican government, the company also managed four ships for TMM Line—Transportacions Maritimas Mexicanos—called *Amparo*, *Elena*, *Samia* and *Josefa*. In total, there were 16 ships in the company's control, with the 12 wholly owned ships having British officers and Indian crew, and the four managed ships having British officers and British, or British-Somalian, crew.

Reardon Smith only carried dry cargo, like coal, grain, molasses, etc., and steel, timber and wood pulp, plus general cargo that included cars, perfume components, fancy goods, clothing, films, guns or whatever was needed to be transported from one country to another. The company had one dedicated car carrier—the *Indian City*—which was a sister ship to the *Atlantic City*, both of 45,000 tonnes deadweight. In the 1970s the *Indian City* was the largest car carrier in the world, regularly carrying 4,000 cars from Japan to Mexico. Unlike today's car carriers, where the cars are driven on, the *Indian City* had to lift each car on by derricks[3] and each car would then be driven into its position inches away from the car in front. The vessel had seven holds and about 12 decks per hold. The loading and unloading were a frenzy of work and it was possible to load 4,000 cars individually in just 24 hours!

So it was, at the end of his leave, Michael joined the *MV Atlantic City* at the Bunge Grain Terminal in Rotterdam, where she was loading grain for New Orleans in America. Upon meeting up with the other officers, his stomach fell. The catering officer was the very same chap from his first ship, who not only knew Michael's weaknesses, but also those dreaded names they used to call him. It got worse before it got better. Because the vessel wasn't quite on the berth when the officers arrived, they were put up in a nearby hotel overnight. Perhaps the accommodations officer had thought that the two officers from the same ship would like to share one of the twin rooms. They couldn't have been more wrong. Landed with Officer A, he and Michael barely spoke all night, which suited Michael just fine.

The next day dawned with more positive news, and relief for Michael. Upon boarding the new vessel, he found that there was only one other cadet on board, and it was his first trip. As the more senior cadet, Michael, enjoyed his perceived position of power!

---

3 A type of marine crane.

The Sea gods were certainly smiling on Michael for his second voyage, as the captain was only 28, and as the youngest captain in the company, he was much nearer in age to Michael, whilst his boss, the chief officer, RS, had his wife, S, with him. They were all such nice people that Michael became lifelong friends with RS and S, regularly going to their house in Devon when he was at naval college in Plymouth.

Chapter 6

Let the Good Times Roll (and Pitch)

THE *MV ATLANTIC CITY* was a 45,000 deadweight bulk carrier with seven cargo holds, all forward of the accommodation. She was around 700 feet long. The cargo holds were about 50 feet deep, and the only way to get to the bottom was down a vertical ladder—all the way down with no platforms to rest at on the way up or down.

The ship sailed from Rotterdam, across the North Atlantic Ocean, around the coast of Florida and into and up the Mississippi River to New Orleans. The berth in NOLA,[4] as New Orleans is known, was not ready, and the ship had to anchor up in a holding anchorage about five miles downriver from the main NOLA berths. Advised by the agent acting for the ship that they would

---

4 New Orleans Louisiana.

be at anchor for four or five days, the captain allowed everyone to go ashore as long as they could get back for midnight. Clearly a kindly captain, he also agreed that he would stay on watch, thereby letting all the deck officers—first, second and third officers—have some time off; plus most of the engineers were allowed to go as well, leaving just the second engineer to run the ship. This is a rare situation, as ships at anchor still have to maintain a deck and engine room watch 24/7 for safety reasons. It is quite rare for a captain to agree to do almost 12 hours of continuous watch-keeping without an officer to support him.

Nonetheless, it was agreed that 90 per cent of the officers would take some time out, and a launch was arranged for 1600 hours to ferry them all to the town berth in NOLA. They split up into small groups and inevitably ended up in the French Quarter and Bourbon Street where they regrouped. At the time there was a famous Irish bar called Pat O'Brien's in the Bourbon Street area that served pitchers of beer and cocktails. It was a jolly drinking hole which often had a musician, and if you bought a pitcher of beer they gave you a polystyrene straw boater to wear as you swayed in time to the music.

To comply with the captain's instructions to be back by midnight, Michael and his shipmates ordered several taxis to take them all back to the boat jetty to get the ferry back. As the big powerful engines roared into life and they headed down river, Michael reflected on what a good time had been had by all. Some more so than others! With the chief officer—also known as the first officer—and his wife, as well as the chief engineer and his wife, in the party, they naturally took responsibility for getting everyone back as per the captain's instruction, but were in for a big surprise. The ship had gone!

Shocked and intrigued, the ferry radioed port control to find out where the ship was and learnt that it was heading upriver to its grain berth as a space had become available. But how could that be? thought Michael and the rest of the revellers, as there weren't any deck officers or engineers on board except for a skeleton crew. There was only the captain to run the bridge—plus the Indian crew—and to steam upriver would require the captain and an officer. Also, there was only one engineer plus crew on board, and it required two people to run the engine for safety reasons. How on earth, they wondered, was the ship going to tie up alongside, as it required an officer and crew in the bows, and an officer and crew at the stern. It was all very puzzling, but they decided they would find out soon!

Ferried to the landing point, they asked for a bus to take them back to the ship. This simple request created two more problems for the now somewhat peeved party-goers. Firstly, the ship hadn't arrived so they couldn't travel there, and then secondly, the earliest they could get a bus was at 7 am—six hours away! With little money left, and absolutely no chance of getting a hotel room, they decided to walk the streets of New Orleans until one of the engineers suggested they sleep on the wide central reservation of an eight-lane highway. It seemed like a good idea until a police car stopped and told them to move on or they would be arrested for jay walking! They had no choice then but to find a quiet area and sit on the ground counting the hours until at 7 am. A school bus picked them up and drove them the five miles upriver to the grain elevator, where their ship, the *Atlantic City*, had mysteriously berthed. They were greeted by banners across the gangway welcoming them home, put up by the captain, proving that he was not only a nice guy, but also a comedian; and although they were all exhausted, they could see the funny side of it. He proved his very worthy credentials even more when he agreed to keep the deck watch overseeing the discharge of the grain for four hours, allowing those due to go on watch the chance to get a little sleep.

Technically, missing the ship when it is due to depart is a serious offence and a man could be 'logged' for it. This is where his name is entered into the ship's log book with a record of his 'crime', meaning that once the owners saw who had been logged, they had the right to dismiss him from service. On this occasion the captain let it pass. Most of the returning revellers found this to be a great relief, but for the chief officer and chief engineer, it was a bit embarrassing.

Having discharged part of the cargo in NOLA, the ship continued on to Vera Cruz in Mexico to discharge the rest. Facilities in Mexico for discharging thousands of tonnes[5] of grain were nowhere near as sophisticated as they had been in NOLA where they used grabs on the end of cranes to pick up about 50 tonnes of grain at a time. The Mexican grabs, when they worked, could only lift a tenth of that amount, so it meant that the ship would be in harbour for two to three weeks.

When the captain allowed some of the crew to take one of the lifeboats to a deserted beach, Michael really appreciated just how different and wonderful it was to be on this ship compared to the *Welsh City*. Spotting the sailors having a barbecue on the beach, the locals turned up with a team of horses and offered them rides for a reasonable price. Though fearful, Michael allowed himself to be cajoled into joining in and asked the handler for a gentle

---

5 A tonne is a metric ton of 1,000 kg, as opposed to a ton which is 20 cwt or 2,240 lbs.

horse. The phrase 'beware of Greeks bearing gifts' could well be changed to 'beware of Mexicans offering gentle horses' here, as that was, of course, exactly what Michael did not get! Instead his horse was given a good thwack on its rump and bolted off with poor Michael, half out of his saddle, hanging on for dear life. Though everyone else thought this was incredibly funny, the rider was more terrified than amused and wonders how he managed not to soil himself! Eventually, the horse stopped and the laughter died down and Michael asked the handler what had happened to the quiet horse he'd requested.

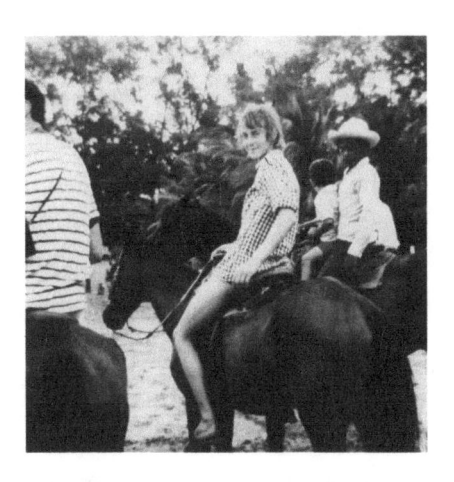

My beach horse ride (MV Atlantic City)

"There's no such thing as a quiet horse," he was told, so accepting that he would never be at ease around horses, he did try to see the funny side of things.

Back on board, Michael in his senior cadet role was waiting for first-timer, JC, to join him at the bottom of the hold. Some sixth sense made him look up, where to his horror he saw a bucket of tools hurtling its way towards his head. Fortunately, he managed to move out of the way in the nick of time as it crashed onto the floor with a mighty clang. Realising that he could just have been very seriously injured, or indeed killed, he asked JC what he was up to, and upon hearing that the bucket had got knocked over the edge accidently, he felt a sliver of fear shiver up his spine. There is no edge around the hole where the ladder goes through the deck;

instead, it is protected by a 10-inch coaming, or lip, and for the bucket to have come down the hole base first was not possible. It could only have done so deliberately. Michael reported the incident to the chief officer, who agreed that it was probably an accident, but Michael knew differently. He was, from that moment, very guarded around his subordinate cadet, never allowing himself to be in a position where he could come to harm.

They say that karma takes care of the things that are unjust, and it certainly sounds as though JC got his comeuppance in the end. On his next ship he showed his true colours when drunk one evening he sat on the rails at the stern. When the ship took a sudden lurch, he fell backwards into the sea without anyone noticing. It wasn't until he failed to turn up for work at nine the next morning that the alarm was raised. His whereabouts could only be verified up until 12 hours earlier, so after calculating the ship's position at that time, a message was sent out to all ships that a man was overboard. With the area known for having sharks and killer whales, time was of the essence, and JC was extremely lucky to be picked up by a British cargo ship. The worse for wear but still alive, he became a minor celebrity when the media got hold of the story of his survival against the odds, but once that had all calmed down, he was unceremoniously sacked from the company for being such an idiot!

In the 1970s Mexico was still an underdeveloped country, and this was quite apparent when you walked into town in Vera Cruz. Small shanty-style shops sold everything you could possibly imagine and at its centre was the square with its bars, fruit cocktail bar and mariachi bands touting for money. Whilst many of Michael's shipmates went into town in search of a bar to drink in, his choice was to sit in the shade in the centre and drink a fruit cocktail or have an ice cream. He never saw any point in drinking to excess, and still doesn't.

In Mexico at that time, the average weekly income of the locals was very low and they could not afford the luxuries that were enjoyed on board ship. Sailors were given bars of Lux or Camay soap to shower with—untold riches to the Mexicans.

So it was one evening that some 'ladies' boarded the *MV Atlantic City* selling their bodies. As a 17-year-old virgin this was, Michael realised, his opportunity to lose his virginity. Finding that he didn't have enough American dollars, the currency preferred to pay his working girl, she happily accepted two bars of soap in exchange for his cherry.

After three weeks or so in Vera Cruz, Michael's second voyage, so full of good times, came to an end in Rotterdam from whence he returned to college to continue his training.

Chapter 7

A First Time for Everything

WITH 10 DAYS' LEAVE before he would return to college in Plymouth, Michael decided it was time to ditch public transport and get his own set of wheels. With his dad's help he bought his first motor: a Morris Minor 1000, four-door saloon, which at 13 years old was by no means shiny and new— but it worked and it was all his. Being such a car enthusiast, he can still remember the registration plate: 103 BGP. One wonders if it is still around today.

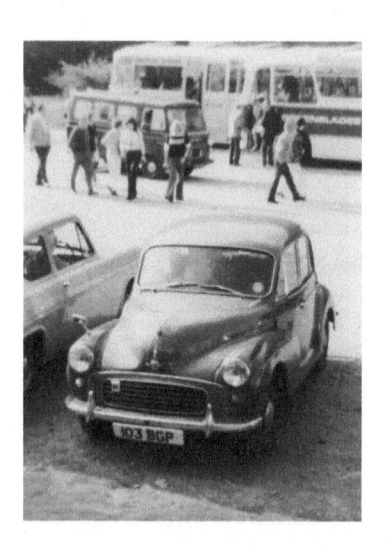

My 1st car - Morris Minor 1000

With no motorway links in 1973, the drive to Plymouth via the A38 was, shall we say, scenic. Taking Michael eight hours from the East Midlands, he was relieved to arrive at the familiar Plymouth School of Maritime Studies' halls of residence where, just as he had suspected, everything was the same: the same morning wake-up call, delivered by the very same navy petty officer.

Though the name of his roommate is lost in the ether, Michael recalls that he had plenty of friends—though it might be more accurate to say that his car had plenty of 'friends'! That said, he'd remained pals with many of the cadets he'd met on his earlier induction course, so having the car was a bonus in terms of social gratification. Petrol in 1973 was rationed due to the oil crisis, so even if he'd been able to afford it, he wouldn't have been able to drive out to explore areas outside of Plymouth, but having a ride out to the local shopping area, Ernesettle Sports Centre and the marine site were his limit.

Not being a beer drinker, weekend nights out with the lads were pretty much off Michael's agenda; instead he decided to widen his social life by getting involved with activities and clubs in the local area. The Plympton Small Bore Rifle Club caught his eye. On his first visit, he was picked up from his residence by the club manager, PS, and driven to the rifle club. Housed in a long, single-storey building, he was met by the sight of other members shooting their 22-bullet rifles and was keen to have a go. After being shown how best to lie on the floor and support his gun, he was ready to fire. Though he hit the target but missed the bull's eye, his shot had gone home and he quickly signed up to be a formal member of the club. Every Tuesday P would pick him up in his Austin 1300, then they'd shoot a few rounds and pop a few more in the local pub. With practice, Michael's skills improved and he was placed in the 'B' team, taking part in competitions with other clubs. Though there were many contests, the one which sticks in his mind the most is when they competed against the Citadel army barracks team in Plymouth and won. It was a great feeling to beat a team who shot rifles for a living!

In 1973 bisexuality was still illegal for men under the age of 21—and then it was only permitted in private. Aged 18, Michael knew he was bisexual so, being careful, decided to explore some of the lesser-known nightspots of Plymouth. He took his first foray into gay society when he paid to go into a nightclub at the top of the Hoe one Saturday night. He ended up talking with two men who were, insofar as they could be within the law, a couple. Three turned into four when they were joined by KL, and Michael's social and sexual life became very interesting.

At 30, KL was a lot older than Michael, but after going to the couple's house for coffee and feeling safe and comfortable with his companions, Michael ended up sleeping with his new older friend. KL was a kind and gentle guy and their lovemaking was exquisite. Michael became very fond of him.

Knowing that he'd been out all night, Michael's room mates were very curious as to where he'd been. Though their pestering for information was in its own way delightful, Michael was honour bound by loyalty and law not to whisper a word. Apart from that, homosexuality at the time was considered a criminal offence in the Merchant Navy, so he had far more to lose than his dignity. He wanted to keep his career as well as his freedom, so with it being his life and his story, it remained his secret.

Meeting up with KL the following weekend at the same club, he suggested they go back to his place at the end of the night. Walking along the car-lined street, Michael was astonished to find himself looking at the personal plates of a Rolls Royce Silver Cloud—the plates themselves would've cost at least £600 back then—but feeling easy in KL's company, Michael slid into the passenger seat and relaxed back into the luxury of the Rolls. By the time they arrived at KL's second home, a comfortable bungalow at the end of a mile-long single-track road, Michael had learned that his lover owned and dealt in property in London and owned several hotels in the local area. Arriving at the charming home in such luxury, Michael had no reason to doubt him. Their relationship lasted the length of Michael's four-month tenure at college, but sadly they lost touch when he went back to sea.

Where one older chap was warm and kind, another was cool and strict. He had to be: he was Chiefy T—ex-Royal Navy yeoman of signals and the course signals tutor—and it was his job to get his young seamen through their exams. Whilst his methods were not liked, and therefore Michael didn't much like the man, he knew deep down that Chiefy T was doing exactly what he needed to. Learning chartwork, all manner of signals including the meaning of different flags, morse code and semaphore was no walk in the park, and when it was your turn to be picked on to answer a question, the chief made you sweat until you got it right. He was a good tutor and his methods worked—Michael and his classmates all passed their exams. Learning about the cosmos—stars, constellations, planets and the rotation of the sun and moon—was much more interesting, but when there was nothing more to do the cadets were allowed to go swimming. Being a non-swimmer, Michael was given lessons, and although he only had two during phase one of his training, he wasn't worried. He still couldn't swim, but neither could he fly, and going in aeroplanes didn't faze him, so neither did being on board a ship.

Named after a port in Vancouver Island, Western Canada, where it regularly called in to load wood pulp, Michael's next ship was the *MV Port Alberni City*. It was recognisable for the 10-foot-high lettering of 'CELTIC BC' painted on each side of its hull. Celtic Bulk Carriers was a shared contract with Irish Shipping Line Ltd, and both companies loaded timber products and packaged wood pulp in Western Canadian ports for discharge in Europe. It was a world away from the malodorous molasses of Michael's first ship and ghastly grain of the second.

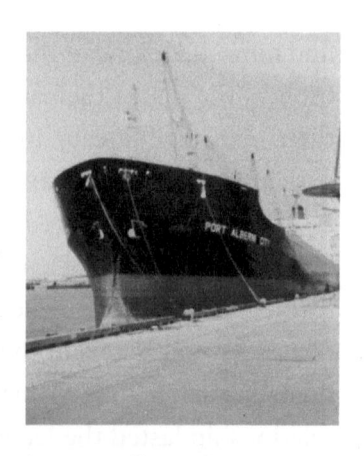

MV Port Alberni City

The *Port Alberni City* was a 25,000 deadweight bulk carrier of about 600 feet in length. She had five holds with no tween decks. Towering above each hold was a 15 tons lifting capacity Hagglund hydraulic crane. The cargo holds were covered in motorised MacGregor hatch covers which could be bolted down onto the hatch coamings to keep the cargo free of the damp sea air and the weather. The company had a few of this type of vessel, as they were ideally suited to the Celtic BC contract.

Like most ships of this time, the accommodation was aft and included an open-air swimming pool. The pool could be filled with seawater and measured about 20 feet by 10 feet and around six to eight feet deep. It was situated on one of the upper decks just behind the funnel.

To dispel the ideas that many people have, the ship's funnel isn't an oversized chimney, but it did have the engine exhaust pipes. The funnel would be about 12 feet in diameter with two

16-inch exhaust pipes running through to the top which belched smoke. There was a steel catwalk inside the funnel and a ladder going down into the engine room. Funnels didn't need to be so big, but they were the ideal way to display the company's branding, and Reardon Smith Lines' was a large black 'S' on a pillar-box-red background.

In front of the funnel was the navigation bridge which spanned the entire width of the ship, with the wheelhouse stretching across to each side of the accommodation block and the bridge wings continuing to the extreme edges each side.

When at sea, the wheelhouse would be in the charge of the officer of the watch who would be supported by an Indian lookout. The ship's watches were divided equally between the three navigation officers—the third officer taking the 8 pm to 12 midnight watches, the second officer the 12 midnight to 4 am watches and the chief officer the remaining 4 to 8 am watches. The structure of each day meant it was impossible to get more than about six hours' continuous sleep.

In addition to the watches, each officer had responsibilities on deck. The third mate was in charge of the lifesaving equipment and its maintenance, the second mate the firefighting equipment plus maintaining all the navigation charts and publications together with plotting all courses for each voyage, and the chief mate was in control of all of the ship and the ship's crew, with the exception of the engine room.

Each week it was a requirement to carry out a fire and emergency drill. Usually at around 0900 hours on a Saturday morning the captain would take over the bridge and the ship's fire alarms sounded. All officers and crew then had to don their lifejackets and safety helmets and present at the lifeboat muster points on each side of the accommodation. The lifeboats were designed to be able to take all of the ship's complement, but for the purpose of drills each lifeboat was attended by half of the crew on each side.

Once the lifeboat roster had been completed and all lifejackets observed to be worn correctly, the alarm bells would ring again to signal a 'fire' and the crew would attend a pretend fire at some part of the ship. Fire hoses would be run out and tested, a 'body' would be found and the flexible stretcher deployed to retrieve the body and return to the accommodation with the six crewmen carrying the stretcher. Once the lifeboat and fire drills were completed, the captain made an entry in the ship's official logbook and the third mate resumed his task of being the officer on the bridge.

Michael found the drills to be very routine and in hindsight thought they could have been made more demanding and more rewarding. When he returned as a safety inspector contracted by various shipping companies, his hum-drum experiences led him to make the fire and safety drills much more realistic, and thus exciting.

Having joined the *Port Alberni* in Antwerp where it was discharging its cargo, Michael had several days in dock to make an impression on his fellow officers who were already on board. It didn't take him long, as he arrived wearing a leather jacket, black skintight trousers with a pink leg seam and platform shoes. Michael thought he looked cool. They thought he looked queer!

Within a couple of days he was invited to join some of his colleagues on a night out to enjoy some of Antwerp's seedy bars. Seeing this as a good opportunity to be 'one of the lads', he decided to go. One of the many bars they went into was Danny's, infamous amongst seafarers in the 1970s as being a welcoming place for transvestites to frequent. Michael was warned that the 'women' weren't really female, but he didn't care. He got talking to a 'girl' in her 20s and ended up taking her back to his cabin. From then on the other officers were convinced he was gay, and since trying to tell them that the girl wasn't actually a man only made him look stupid, he didn't bother. The bullying and humiliating behaviour he had experienced as a first-time, naïve cadet resurfaced, though this time it was because he was thought to be gay. At least this time the captain, and a small number of other people, treated him properly.

Though this was his first trip on the *MV Port Alberni City*, it would not be his last. His seaman's discharge book reliably informs him he joined the ship on 20 February 1974 and was paid off in Corpus Christi, Texas, USA, four months later on 14 June, when he went on three months' paid leave. Though he remembers that the captain was a pleasant Irishman by the name of T McN, the voyage itself could not have been very remarkable, as he has few memories of it other than making an impression and being sexually misunderstood. His one other clear memory is of the ship's electrician, who stands out as being a big chap—he was as tall as he was wide.

The *Port Alberni City*, together with her sister ships, *Vancouver City*, *Prince Rupert City*, *Fresno City*, *Victoria City* and *Tacoma City*, were built by Upper Clyde Shipbuilders of Glasgow between 1970 and 1972. They were all 570 feet long and 83 feet 6 inches wide, and when fully loaded they had 33 feet 6 inches below the water line. The engines were Burmeister & Wain 6-cylinder K-type engines producing 11,600 BHP. Their service speed was 15.5 knots (nautical miles per hour, where 1 nautical mile is 6,080 feet) and they consumed 36 tons of oil per day. They were all registered in Bideford, Devon.

Chapter 8

Japanese Japes

MICHAEL BOARDED HIS NEXT SHIP in Rotterdam. The *MV New Westminster City* was similar in style to the *Port Alberni City*, and just like his first trip on that vessel, was an unremarkable voyage, except that it was the first time that he was able to welcome his family aboard. Discharging a cargo of steel in Immingham, his mum, dad and sister, Linda, went to see him and were given a tour of the ship. His dad was most impressed with the bridge. Paying off on 15 April 1973, and after a short period of leave, he once again headed back to Plymouth for further training.

Having sold his Morris Minor but still wanting to be independent, Michael bought his next car off someone his dad knew for the princely sum of £25. Though big and heavy, he was very happy with his new Morris Oxford and was proud that it didn't look out of place amongst the Ford Anglia 100E and a Zephyr Six in the car park of his new college residence.

Unlike the dormitories of his first accommodation, this new place was a hall of residence situated in a two-storey Victorian building with about 30 individual rooms. The wake-up call was also unlike that of the previous lodgings—not an indiscretion to be heard. This time the manager was a down-to-earth chap who, with the aid of his wife, ran a relaxed regime with regular meals and events for the cadets to join in with. So it was one Saturday evening at an organised disco that Michael hooked up with a local girl. Being suave and sophisticated, and of course not wanting to be indiscrete either, instead of taking her back up to his room, he took her to, and in, her Mini Countryman instead. On another occasion at a disco in the residence of some trainee nursery nurses, Michael behaved in a much more sophisticated manner when plucking up the courage to talk to the only other person not dancing; he accepted an invitation to see her at her parents' house in Dartmoor the following weekend. It was the beginning of his long relationship with JW.

Though he passed his second mate exams in 1975, Michael failed his radar certificate. Trained on two radars held in premises up on Plymouth Hoe, he was also 'put in charge' of simulated ships sailing up the English Channel on a radar simulator. Having to use his radar skills to negotiate numerous other 'targets' on the radar, Michael decided not to take his supertanker up the English Channel as instructed, but instead brought his ship into Plymouth. He didn't go around the breakwater, but chose instead to drive his ship over it and 'parked' it in the fishing boat berths. Whilst his mates thought this was awfully funny, his tutor did not, so he paid the price for being the class clown by failing his exam. He couldn't take up his promotion to third officer[6] on his next ship

---

[6] The system is that the third mate has a second mate's certificate, and all ranks have the next certificate above their rank.

either. Instead, he was promoted to fourth officer. Pleased that he had received a promotion, he phoned JW to tell her the good news, confiding that he thought he might get a pay rise that would take him up to £40 per week, so he was pleasantly surprised when he got nearly £100 per week instead.

He joined his fourth ship, the *MV Indian City*, on 2 January 1976 at New Westminster in British Columbia, Canada. The 45,000 deadweight car carrier had a long-term contract with Datsun (now known as Nissan) to take cars to the USA and Mexico. Though he doesn't recall loading cargo for the return trip to Japan, he does remember that he got on very well with his shipmates—so much so that he nearly ended up in prison!

Docked in Nagoya with empty holds and 4,000 cars on the quay ready to be loaded, Michael, the radio officer and the chief steward all went ashore to a bar and—unusually for him—got a bit merry with his friends. On walking back to the ship, they decided to go for a joy ride up and down the quay in one of the waiting cars. As each car was allowed one gallon of petrol to enable them to be driven to the ship and to be driven away from the ship on arrival in the USA, they all clambered into a Datsun Cherry and started to have some fun.

Not content with the baby-sized Datsun Cherry, Michael swapped to a sporty Datsun 260Z, and when he ran out of fuel just left it where it stopped and got into another one. Why not? he thought; there were thousands to play in! After driving this second car around the quay he noticed a police car coming towards him with its lights flashing. Though he didn't think it was coming for him, as it was going so slow, he stopped his car, then noticed that his two friends had debussed and were running back to the gangway and back on board the ship. With the police car still trundling towards him, he thought he should perhaps do the same. With a growing sense that all was not well, he searched for the door handle, not realizing that on that type of sports car it lies next to the seat cushion, so he wound down the window and tried to climb through. That didn't work, but somehow in his efforts he managed to open the door and pegged it back in a very unsteady line back to the ship, up the gangway and into his cabin, where he hastily undressed and dived into bed, thinking that if he was 'fast asleep' when his door was opened, he would appear less likely to be the guilty party.

Not having to get up early the next day, it was mid morning when, on his way to the galley to get his first coffee, he was told the captain wanted to see him. With his gut tightening, he made his way to find out just how much shit had hit the fan. Captain RS's first words to him were, "Somebody was driving cars up and down the quay last night. Was it you?" From the tone of his voice, Michael knew fine well that he had no doubts that it was, so he owned up straight away. Captain RS then went on to explain that the police hadn't come on board following the incident, but had waited until the ship had woken up and had then interrogated the captain at 0800 hours, explaining that three people had been driving cars on the dock and that it was a criminal offence in Japan to do so, punishable with a heavy fine and up to two years in prison. Clearly in shock, the captain had replied that he knew that none of his officers or crew would do such a thing, and when the police stated that the culprits had got on board at around 0400 hours, the captain replied that they must have just taken refuge on the ship and would have climbed down a rope to the jetty when the police weren't looking. Whether they believed him or not, they accepted the explanation and left.

Not knowing what to say, Michael stayed silent but was expecting to be in trouble, at least, with his captain for the previous night's drama. He was told there and then what a stupid thing it had been to do and that the captain wouldn't be logging him, as when he was a younger officer, he had done the very same thing! The next day and night it was noticeable just how visible the police were, but the culprits didn't show themselves again!

When cars are loaded into each deck level, they are driven to within two inches of the car loaded before them, so that the passenger door is blocked but the driver's door is clear to open. The decks are only six feet apart, so whilst it is possible to walk in the spaces where there are no cars, it is impossible to move around the cars when each deck has been filled. To allow the crew to move around the decks they had to crawl across the bonnets of each car, for which Datsun issued them with soft trainers to wear instead of the steel-toecap shoes they would normally wear.

Once a deck was full of cars, the portable deck plates that filled the central hole above were then lowered into place by the stevedores and securely fixed. However, on some occasions the descending deck plates would miss their fixings and crush the 20 or so cars beneath them. Whilst this may appear to be a costly mistake, Datsun still sent the damaged cars to their destination, where the top of the cars, from the waistline upwards, were cut off and new 'tops' welded into place. Knowing this, Michael has never ever purchased a Datsun.

With such a good crowd on board, Michael thoroughly enjoyed his time on the *Indian City*. The last voyage on this ship was to take Datsun cars and pick-ups to Jeddah in the Red Sea. The passage round from Japan meant stopping off for stores and fuel in Singapore. As Singapore was well known for 'bum boats'—little skiffs with people wanting to come on board to steal what they could find—Michael was tasked with standing on the top of the gangway to dissuade these people from coming on board. Some of the crew were not too pleased with him though, as they wanted to buy some of the cheap watches these bum boats often had for sale. However, he was true to his task, and not one person was allowed on board unless they had official business.

Their voyage ended in the anchorage area of Jeddah, where they found about one hundred other ships all waiting to unload their cargoes. At that time Jeddah was a developing port, and the Saudi rulers were buying up cargo from all sorts of countries. Other ships had general cargo, fruit, oil, Coca-Cola, camels and—like the *Indian City*—vehicles. The fruit ships were on a tight deadline because the fruit couldn't be kept fresh for too long before it would start to go off. The port authorities allowed ships to dock based upon how important their cargoes were, and bananas weren't considered a priority. Instead, the ship carrying Coca-Cola was allowed to discharge first, followed by the camels, then the vehicles. Whilst the crews on the fruit ships took to their lifeboats to deliver the fruit to the other ships as they didn't want it to go to waste, Michael also left the *Indian City*, just three months after he joined it, on 9 April 1976.

Chapter 9

Scares and Successes

UPON HIS RETURN HOME from the *Indian City*, Michael had to resit his radar certificate and enjoy some leave. As a cadet, he'd had one week's leave per month served on board, but as an officer leave was doubled, so he was effectively working two on, one off. Given his previous failure, it might be hard to pass his radar exam, but enjoying some leave would be easy.

He enrolled on a radar course with the London Polytechnic's Tower Bridge Centre as soon as he arrived home. Unlike Plymouth, that used a static radar facility, the London crowd used a converted minesweeper—the Sir John Cass—belonging to The Marine Society. This was a far more realistic arrangement and was a good shout going up and down the River Thames. Thankfully, the three-week course culminated in him passing the exam, and he was finally promoted to third officer by the company.

He joined his next ship, the *MV Vancouver City*, in Singapore on 8 August 1976 as third mate and embarked on a fairly unmemorable journey, apart, that is, from his experience in the Bermuda Triangle.

Voyaging back to Europe from the Gulf of Mexico, the ship had sailed the coastal route around the Florida Keys and was heading out into the Atlantic Ocean. As third officer, Michael was on watch from 8 pm to midnight. Around 9.30 pm, and already dark, he was standing about six feet back from the forward-facing bridge windows, keeping a general eye on the waters ahead, when a bright light caused the shadows of the window frames to go from the back of the bridge to the front. It lit up all of the windows, so was either a very close light—like 100 feet above the ship—or a very bright light further away.

Michael's first thought was that it must have been an aircraft in distress, so he rushed to the bridge wing, but there was nothing visible. He ran back to the radar, which has a good response on the 24-mile radius, or a reasonable response on a 48-mile range, but there was nothing. If it were an aircraft, he reasoned, it couldn't have flown 48 miles in a few seconds, and if it had ditched, the resultant waves from the impact would have shown on the radar. But there was nothing. Actually, he thought, there hadn't been any sound either. So . . . what was it? Michael called the captain, who like him checked the radar and the horizon. He agreed with Michael. There was nothing to see. He told Michael to carry on keeping the lookout and to call him immediately if the same thing happened again.

That's just great, Michael thought as he realised that the ship was in the middle of the Bermuda Triangle —a notorious spot for planes and ships to suddenly disappear off the face of the earth!

To say he was bricking it would be an understatement; he had after all just had a really weird and unnerving experience on a ship in the Bermuda Triangle! There was nothing else for it though, so he locked both bridge-wing doors (maybe to keep him safe from aliens?) and spent the final two hours of his watch scared witless, waiting for some spaceship to steal them all away.

His six-month voyage paid off in Dublin on 3 February 1977, but the excitement didn't end quite there. Having packed his suitcase the night before, when he arrived at Dublin airport he was surprised when the case set the alarms off. Enquiring what the problem was, he was told by security that his case had triggered the explosives alarm!

Michael knew his case had not been tampered with and he certainly wasn't smuggling explosives, so he accepted that security would go through all his stuff, because he knew they wouldn't find anything. After he'd repacked he was asked if he had had his laundry done just before he'd packed his case on board. He confirmed that he had and was shocked and interested to hear that the detergents used in some laundries can cause a small amount of 'gas' to build up which can trigger the explosives alarm. Apparently it was not the first time the airport staff had encountered such a problem, but it was certainly a first time for Michael, who somewhat red faced rejoined his colleagues and hastily boarded his plane back to London.

Not needing the money but wanting the distraction of meaningful work whilst on leave, Michael decided to get a temporary job to keep him occupied during the day. He approached the transport department at Kettering General Hospital and asked if there were any driving jobs available. JD, the transport manager and senior ambulance officer, told him they could do with another driver, but they had no budget. Happy to work for nothing—after all, he was being paid by Reardon Smith—JD was quick to say he would check with management what could be done. A couple of days later he phoned to say that they would indeed like Michael to work as a van driver, but the unions insisted that he was paid. Not surprisingly, when JD asked if that would be okay with him, Michael also quickly said yes! He really was rather well chuffed with this new set-up delivering medical supplies around the county for an extra £120 per week after tax. With everyone aware that he was in the Merchant Navy, they were so happy with the arrangement that Michael worked his round almost every leave for four or five years.

His next ship, the *MV Amparo*, was one of the TMM-managed ships. She was a dedicated general cargo ship of around 16,000 deadweight. Her officers' accommodation was upmarket compared to the ships Michael was used to, but the ship was older. This time his cabin was facing forward, on the port side of the ship, whereas on previous ships it had always been on the port side, facing the sea.

He joined the *Amparo* in Kure, Japan, where she was loading all manner of things for discharge in the Pacific coasts of the USA, Mexico and Central America. The officers were very friendly, and there were two or three officers' wives on board. Enjoyment was high on the

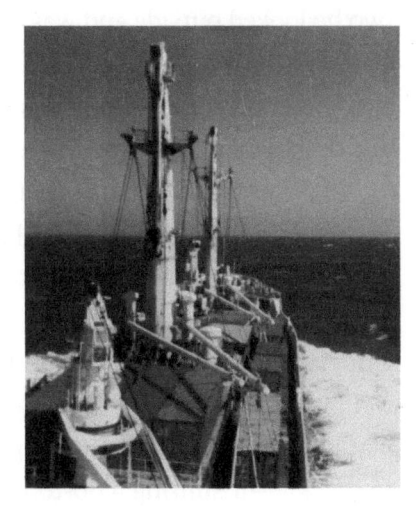

MV Amparo at sea

agenda with quizzes, competitions and lots of social activities, including a 'best legs' competition. Out of all the officers and two of the women, Michael won first prize for having the best legs!

With quite a bit of time spent in Central American ports, Michael particularly remembers one occasion in Costa Rica when he picked up with a girl of ill repute in a bar and went back to her shack for . . .!!!

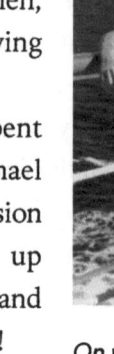

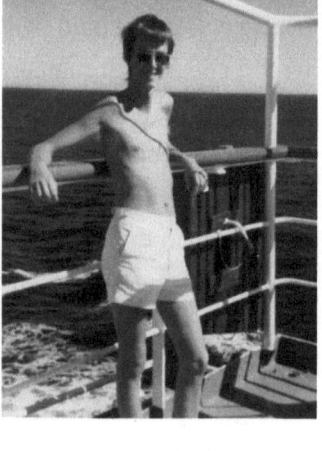

On watch on MV Amparo

Having had a good time, he paid her for her services and decided he ought to get back to the ship, but all he could hear was, he thought, heavy rain. With no coat, he decided to wait for it to stop—only that never happened. So after waiting for an hour or two he looked outside and was dismayed to see that it wasn't rain at all, but the noise of the sea crashing on the shore. His girl's shack was on the beach, and with lust in his eyes he'd failed to notice when he was taken there.

In Nicaragua he recalls that a very heavy road generator that had been shipped over from Japan was on board. It weighed around 60 tons, which wasn't a problem to discharge, as one of their heavy-lift derricks had a capacity of 200 tons. However, whoever had ordered it hadn't done their homework, as the weight on each wheel was too great for the jetty and when it was placed onto it, the structure began to break and the workers had to quickly—if shifting a 60-ton trailer can be done quickly—pull it off the jetty and onto the land.

SCARES AND SUCCESSES

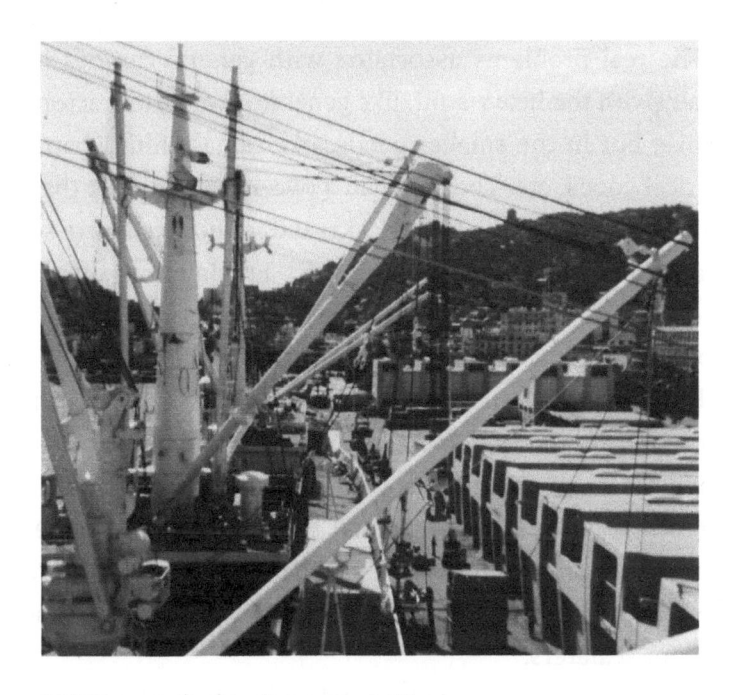

MV Amparo discharging cargo in Mexico

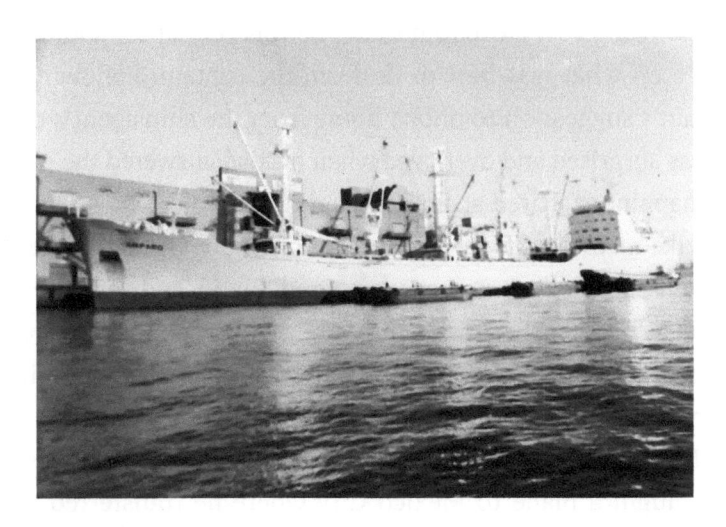

MV Amparo

The real problems associated with general cargoes is not actually with the heavy stuff, like generators or farm tractors and the like, but in the smaller goods, like camera films, batteries, electrical goods, etc. The ship had a tween deck (a deck that was about 20 feet below the main deck), and in this deck were secure storage facilities. No matter how strict a regime was adopted by the captain to stop the stevedores from pilfering, they always found a way to steal some cargo.

Back in Japan Michael decided to go to a gay bar in Kobe he'd found in *The Spartacus Gay Guide*, a handbook of gay bars around the world that he was secretly carrying around with him. He remembers well how kind and friendly the locals were and what a great time he had. It was a shame he couldn't share his experience with his shipmates though, as being gay was still a crime for seafarers.

Happiness turned to sadness when he received a letter from home with news that his dad was in hospital after suffering a heart attack. Being very close to his dad, he was very upset and sought advice on what was best to do from the captain. Following the captain's suggestion to phone home from the ship agent's office, he was surprised and overjoyed when his dad answered the phone. His happiness soared again just hearing his voice.

Like many seafarers, Michael bought some Seiko watches for himself and his dad, as they were good quality and very cheap in Japan. When he gave one to his dad, he was absolutely made up. At least now he'd have a fancy watch to keep time, even if his heart could not.

Michael left the *Amparo* in October 1977 in Guaymas, Mexico, and caught a plane to Mexico City where he transferred to an international flight to Heathrow. Sitting in the middle of three economy-class seats, he got talking with the English lady next to him. They shared tales and stories, and when it came to finding out where they were from, their expressions said it all: what a small world—they were both from Wellingborough!

Chapter 10

No Sex, Please; We're . . .

ARRIVING HOME, MICHAEL GOT STUCK into what would become a regular routine: a week off to recover from his voyage and then back to driving his van for Kettering General Hospital. He bought another stylish car—a Triumph Herald 1200—in which he buzzed around Northamptonshire and popped down to Devon to stay with JW and her family. Taking a bit more time off before joining his next ship, he and JW assured her mum that yes of course they would have separate tents on their trip to the Lake District. They duly packed two—one for them and one for their stores. Propriety was upheld, or at least a semblance of it, in the photos they took of them both allegedly in their own tents, and JW's mum was satisfied that no sex before marriage had gone on!

January 1978 began with the usual phone call advising Michael to make ready to meet his fellow officers and join their next ship, the *Cardiff City* in Gibraltar. Once again nothing about joining a

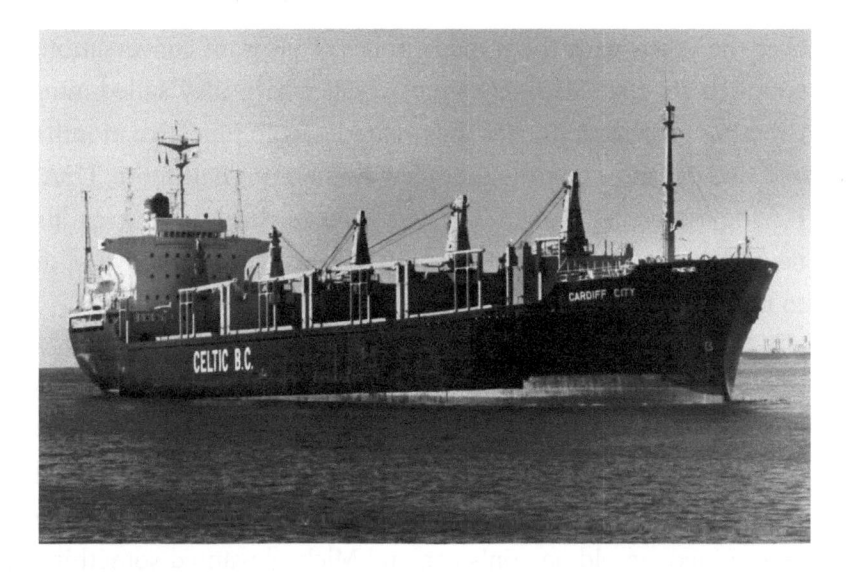

MV Cardiff City

ship was plain sailing, so though they arrived on 22 January ready to board, the ship was still mid Atlantic riding out a storm and wasn't expected until the 25th. Put up in the Hotel Europa, Michael palled up with KS, the radio officer, and one of the engineers. Three days of exploring the island was all they needed to do all the touristy things, including watching the barbary apes, hanging out around the harbour and going underground in the various tunnels. All on full pay. What a life!

The *Cardiff City* was another ship of standard design: a five-hold, five-cranes bulk carrier of 25,000 deadweight. Being a seasoned mariner by now, it held less interest for him than previous ships, so his attention, along with KS's, turned to their shared interest in marine photography. The conversations they had about Michael's new SLR—single lens reflex—camera with zoom and macro lens attachments, and the photos they had both taken over the years, gave them many hours of pleasant conversation; so much so, that Michael cannot recall where they sailed after Gibraltar or what countries they visited. On 26 June, five months and one day after boarding, he flew home from Baltimore, USA. Having a relaxing voyage was just what Michael needed, as his next leave was important. He would be heading back to Plymouth to take his first officer course and exams.

At home he found his dad had upgraded his car, so rather fancying his old one—a Hillman Minx Estate—he gave up the heady days of driving his Triumph Herald and parted with £350 of hard-earned cash for a sensible car. Though it got him to and around Plymouth, he soon realised it just wasn't him. It was, he determined, an old person's car, and Michael wanted something bigger and better. Luckily for him, PG, a DJ at the time on Plymouth Sound, was selling his Vauxhall VX4/90 sports saloon, which Michael snapped up. With its custom paint job similar to that of the famous Starsky & Hutch car, Michael knew it was the one for him. With its rostyle wheels, four headlights, 2.3 litre engine, four gears and two overdrive ratios, it really was the business. Heads certainly turned when he turned up at college in it. Like its new owner, it was fast and impressive.

Although the car occupied his thoughts for much of the time, Michael did manage to knuckle down and get on with his coursework. He passed his exams first time and became the youngest second officer in his company. Fast and impressive, yes; and also wealthier, as his promotion earned him a very welcome pay rise.

Almost a year after leaving the *Cardiff City*, Michael joined the *MV Josefa* in Rotterdam as her second officer. When the crew took his case aboard, the bosun asked if he was a cadet. On being told

NO SEX, PLEASE; WE'RE . . .

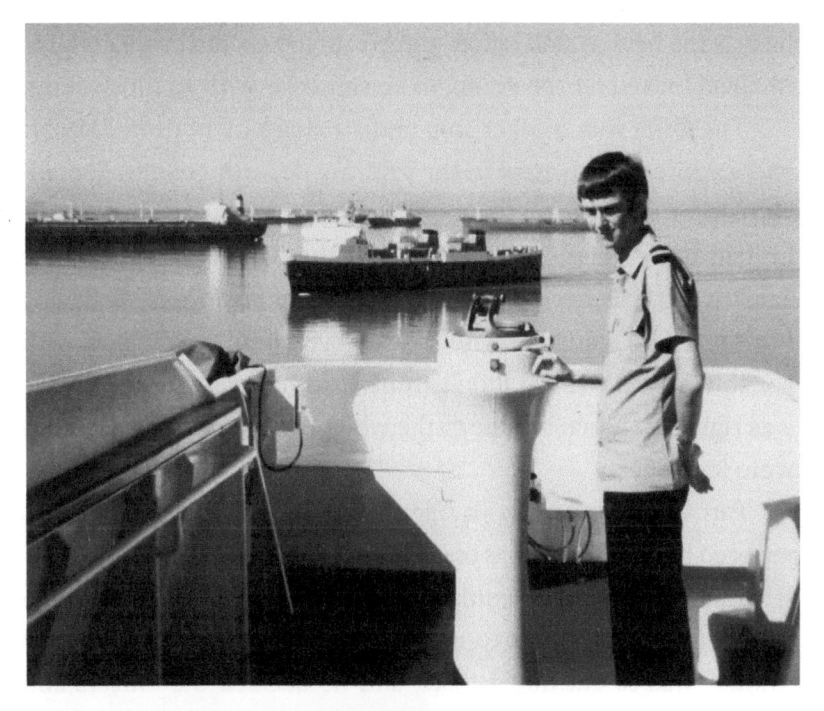

Me as 3rd officer

My Vauxhall VX4/90

he was the new second officer, the bosun took some persuading, as Michael looked far too young to be someone with so much clout.

The *Josefa* was another ship under management from TMM. It had a white-British crew in the catering department and Somali-British for the deck and engine crews. Michael was warned that he had to be careful how he treated the Somali crew, as being sensitive, it was easy to get on the wrong side of them. Believing himself to be someone who treated everyone equally and with consideration, Michael didn't think he'd have any problems. He was right, but when it came to the white British contingent, things were less clear.

Part way through the voyage the captain left the ship and was replaced by a chap who was one of the company's superintendents— JL. This was his first command and he thought he knew best in everything and was out to make a name for himself. One of his 'things' was to cut down costs, and he decided the officers and crew were only allowed three sheets of toilet paper at a time, to save on loo rolls. Michael thought he was a right twat! He then said that engineers could have one bar of soap per week, presumably because they were dirtier, but deck officers were only allowed one bar every two weeks. Needless to say he wasn't well liked for his stupid ideas, and Michael wasn't the only one who had a few choice names for him.

On one occasion Michael remembers that he, SS and PH hired a car to explore the country they were in, though he can't remember which country that was now. They picked the car up the day before and then set out at 8 am the next day. Michael was due on cargo watch at 6 pm and unfortunately the three friends didn't get back until 8 pm, when Michael found that JL had had to do his shift because he'd apparently gone AWOL. When he got on deck the captain ordered him to get his boiler suit on, as he was to take over the cargo watch. Orders or not, Michael was having none of that and told the captain that he hadn't had his required four hours of sleep prior to his shift and so he was going to bed until midnight. A prerequisite of being on watch was that an officer was properly rested beforehand. Aware of this, the captain realised he had no choice but to let Michael have his rest, but his face said much more than any words could have. Michael didn't get logged, but did get a great rollicking from the company.

Having friends like SS, the chief steward, who hailed from Yorkshire, and the captain's steward, PH from Cardiff, made being on the *Josefa* with a disagreeable skipper more than tolerable. It was in fact a voyage of love and laughter. Being quite camp, SS was easy to get on with, and he and Michael had lots in common, though their ideas of how to cut hair differed greatly. Asking him to give him a quick trim one day, Michael had no choice but to go all out for a crew cut after SS deliberately, but only for a laugh, cut his hair into all different shapes and sizes. His relationship with PH was much more effortless. Michael simply fell in love with him. When word spread that he was keen on him, and rumour had it that they sometimes spent time together in Michael's cabin, it didn't take long before one engineer 'nonchalantly' walked past or had a peek through his porthole to see if he could catch them in there.

Michael thought that the *Josefa* was a badly designed ship. The rule of thumb for a ship to be stable at sea was that the breadth had to be one-eighth of the length. So, for example, the *Cardiff City* was 650 feet long and 80 feet wide—fitting the one-eighth rule. The *Josefa* wasn't. Her breadth was less than one-eighth, and as a result she was a cow at sea. She would roll to extremes. Most ships in a swell will roll to around 10 to 15 degrees each way, but the *Josefa* rolled to 25 or 30 degrees each way, meaning that the crew had to use safety lines on deck to stop them falling overboard. Messrooms often saw plates crashing to the deck. It was most unpleasant. She used to have a sister ship, but she was so unstable that she rolled over in port and sank.

Michael remembers that one of the cargoes they loaded was several tonnes of FN automatic rifles plus ammunition. Loaded in Belgium under very tight security, it was destined for the Mexican Navy. On arrival at the port in Mexico, the docks were closed to all traffic; two armed guards were posted on every corner, with many armed navy personnel on board. The guns and ammo were loaded into small trucks the navy had, and as well as the driver and a guard in the cab, two more guards were in the back with the guns. When the last of the dozen trucks had left, the navy commander asked the captain if they could buy some beer from them; it was common knowledge that ships carried several hundred cases of beer at a time. It was agreed to let them have 40 cases, and the truck that carried the beer had six armed guards! Clearly the beer was a more prized cargo than the weapons.

A little after five months, Michael's trip on the *Josefa* ended in Le Havre, France. By then his relationship with JW was over and he had a new girlfriend—a local girl this time—called AT. AT lived about 200 yards from Michael's parents' house, so meeting up was never a problem. Michael got on well with her family: her mum, who was a local councillor, sisters and a brother. Whilst they were together, one of her sisters, and then her brother, joined the Royal Navy as ratings. Michael cannot be sure whether he had a positive or negative influence on their choice of navy.

Although he liked AT a lot, Michael found he just couldn't keep up with her insatiable sex drive. They'd go for a drink but never quite get to the pub, as they'd end up in a quiet lane having sex. It was, Michael remembers, just sex, sex, sex! Which may sound ideal to some, but he actually wanted more out of life than constant bonking. His relationship with JW had ended because he wanted to get engaged and eventually marry, but JW didn't have the same idea. After AT and he had been having sex together for some time, they talked of getting engaged and settling down together, but things went wrong and they parted acrimoniously. At that time neither girl knew that Michael was bisexual. Not that he'd kept it from them: just that it had never come up in conversation. It turned out that AT loved sex so much because she was intent on getting pregnant. Her dream was to have lots of children. Of course, the reason behind Michael's bisexuality would eventually reveal that he would never be able to have children. He could have saved himself the pleasure of all that sex after all!

Chapter 11

I Saw Three Ships...

THREE MONTHS' LEAVE AND driving his van for the hospital led to Michael joining his next vessel. Another ship managed for TMM, this one was called the *MV Samia* and was another general cargo ship, only bigger and, Michael was relieved to find, built to the right proportions.

When you do the same thing month in, month out, it eventually becomes so routine that memories begin to either disappear or not get kept at all because nothing very memorable happens other than the day-to-day running of a big boat. Where the *MV Samia* is concerned, Michael has one very strong memory which, if you're a fan of French perfume, might make you think again about what you dab behind your ears!

Loading honey in Mexico was not such a sticky task, but the part cargo of hefting hessian sacks crammed to the brim with dead flies—yes you read that correctly: dead flies—was an altogether different sort of oppressive assignment. Fifty tons of them completely filled one of the tween decks, and you can imagine the smell. It was as awful, and worse, than your bins being left out over a bank holiday weekend with the temperatures soaring up the thermometer. And who would want sacks full of dead flies anyway? Well, the Parisians: that's who. The dead flies were destined for the French capital, where extracts of them are used to make some high-class perfumes! Yay! Nice smell!! Michael did get the stench out of his nostrils when he disembarked in Le Havre and with a couple of mates took the train to Paris for a free day exploring the city as tourists. Four and a half months after loading the flies, he was once again back home on leave for 10 weeks and another round of hospital driving.

Joining the *Port Alberni City* again, Michael decided not to arrive in his skintight black jeans and platform shoes, though if he had it would have received a different reception, as this time he was with a better set of officers. Landing in Bombay to join the ship, they arrived to find that the ship's agent had organised transport to take them to the port. Taxis? No such luxury. They were piled into the back of a 10-ton, open-backed truck, leaning against the cab whilst their cases acted as seats. As the driver negotiated tight roads congested with a multitude of other drivers and animals, they all just sat back and enjoyed the sun. After all, they were seasoned seafarers, so a bit of bouncing around in high temperatures was nothing new to them.

Much of the time, Michael would wear a boiler suit whilst on deck, but sometimes working in hot weather called for nothing more than a pair of cut-off denims, safety boots and helmet. Nobody thought of skin cancer in those days, so when years later in 2018 Michael developed a lump near his left ear, it was a bit of a shock when his GP thought it could be cancerous due to his exposure to seas of sunshine. Northampton General Hospital were able to assure him it was not malignant, but with that gratefully received gem came the news that because he'd never applied a high-factor suncream whilst at sea, he was now at a higher risk of developing skin cancer in the future. Unlike his first trip on the *Port Alberni*, his second has just melded into more lost or mundane memories. He paid off in Belgium on 10 January 1981, four months after boarding in Bombay.

Back home, Michael decided it was time he got himself a new house. He was after all earning good money, from both his jobs, and living with his parents was just not where he wanted to return after the freedom of the seven seas. He jumped on the housing ladder and eventually bought a three-bed semi on a nice estate in Wellingborough. It was a new definition of 'cool' to be a homeowner, and Michael delved into doing it up just as he wanted it, putting in a new parquet floor in the hall, filling the lounge with vintage or vintage-esque furniture and the bedrooms with, what was at the time, ultra-modern Stag-branded items. Michael's flair for fashion really came out, and he had a great time choosing new dinner sets, cutlery, carpets and the like. Though he no longer wanted to live with them, he was happy for his parents to join in his shopping trips and was delighted to be able to pay his dad for decorating his new place just as he wanted it.

A few years before this his parents had decided to buy the council house they were in and on their accountant's advice were going in for a mortgage. Not happy with that idea, Michael lent them the £6K they needed as an interest-free loan. And though he didn't have the £21,000 he needed to buy his own house outright, he was young and earned a good salary, so was able to put down a good deposit and easily able to afford his own mortgage repayments. Coming home from a few months at sea to an empty house was quite a change from the comfort of his parents' place, but Michael never needed to worry about it being left empty. His old 'mate', BW —the copper who told him off all those years ago for carving his initials into a tree—turned out to be his near neighbour and was happy to keep an eye on things for him.

Next up for Michael was the *Fresno City*, another ship like the *Port Alberni*, with five holds and five cranes with a cargo capacity of

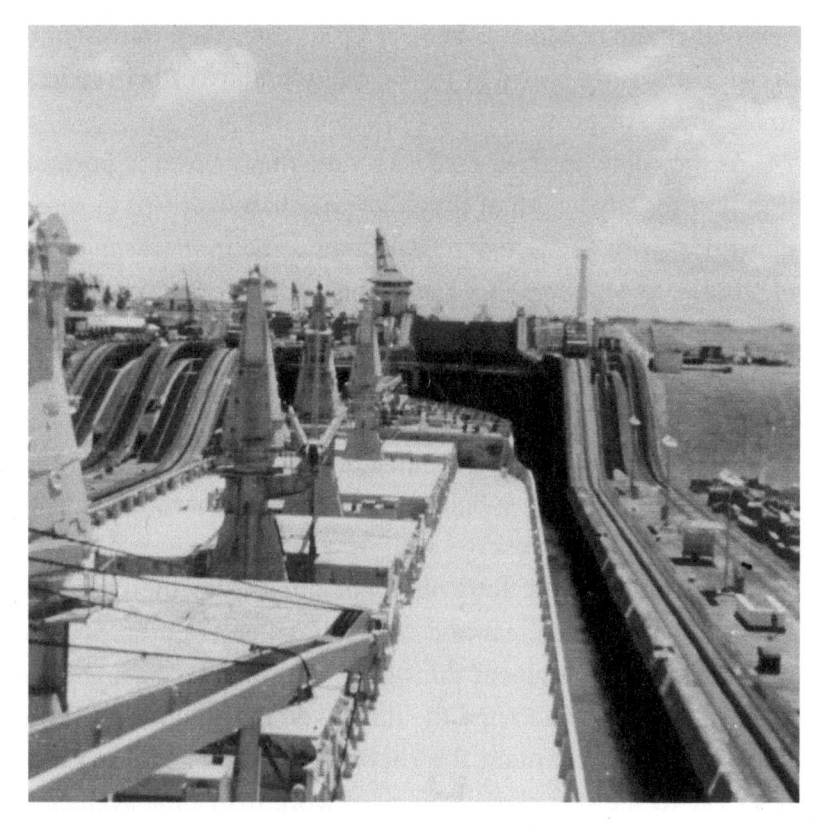

Transiting the Panama Canal

26,000 tonnes deadweight. His record book shows that he joined in Jeddah, Saudi Arabia (in the Red Sea), and left in Rotterdam four months later, on 21 July 1981. He has no lasting memories of the ship, the crew or the voyages.

His duties as second officer were the 12 midnight to 4 am watch, maintenance of the firefighting equipment and the safe navigation of the ship by marking out all the required course lines they needed to follow using the charts held on board. Their chart outfit was for worldwide coverage and constituted around 2,400 individual charts of about three feet by two feet in size. With all charts needing to be kept up to date, they were sent a booklet of updates issued by the British Admiralty, called 'Notices to Mariners', by post.

As they only received mail each time they arrived in port, or if in port for any length of time they may have had two or three deliveries, with each port arrival came some four weeks or so of 'Notice to Mariners' booklets. The number of charts carried that would need amending would run to around 100 to 150 per booklet, and one correction to one chart would take two or three minutes to do properly. One 'N to M' booklet could give Michael seven or eight hours of work updating the charts. Usually they only received four or five booklets at a time, so that was only 30 to 40 hours of extra work!

The watches were four on, eight off, and in the eight off Michael had to sleep, eat and carry out some maintenance on the firefighting equipment during the day, or relax at night. In addition, he also had to find the time to do the 40 hours of extra work needed to maintain the charts to keep them up to date. It's clear to see that there was more work than time available. He couldn't pass his work onto other officers, as they also had more work than time available, so much of his free time was spent updating the charts. Enjoying it as he did, it was not a problem, though most of his colleagues in the fleet hated the chart corrections. Quite often he would join a ship only to find that his predecessor hadn't done the chart maintenance, leaving Michael with several months' work to catch up on.

In maintaining the fire equipment, Michael had to ensure all fire hydrants worked, including the valves and spindles, ensuring the rubber seals inside each hydrant hadn't perished. There were around 25 to 30 hydrants around the ship. He also had to keep the fire mains pipework in good order, which often involved chipping the rust off and repainting with a primer paint and then the bright red topcoat.

The fire extinguishers were also his responsibility, and two of them had to be tested at each weekly fire drill. Michael would then refill and recertify them. He was proficient at refilling dry powder, foam and water extinguishers, but had to send any spent CO_2 extinguishers ashore for refilling. The ship carried two Siebe Gorman fire suits with oxygen tanks, and these also had to be tested each week, and the oxygen topped up to full every time they were used.

On some ships Michael had the responsibility of checking and maintaining the ship's hospital. They had a room dedicated to hospital needs, together with collapsible stretchers, and all the medical supplies and drugs needed to carry out minor operations on board.

During his training he was taught about drug misuse, childbirth and appendectomies, which, if necessary, were operations that could be performed on board if the ship were thousands of miles from immediate help. His work experience at Kettering General

Hospital unfortunately didn't help with his hospital work on board ship!

Life at sea sounds like a good, cushy job, but as Michael warns, "It's long hours and hard." If you don't mind long hours and getting four hours' sleep twice a day, there are good opportunities for people seeking a career at sea, but Michael goes on to counsel, "Just check in with yourself and ask if you are prepared for the unusual hours and constant hard work."

Michael freely admits that his career didn't start well, but he is eternally grateful to his parents for cajoling him into doing his second trip, as by and large he enjoyed his time at sea. Going to different corners of the world, seeing sights he wouldn't ordinarily get to see and meeting some really nice people was very rewarding.

Chapter 12

Watch Out!

HEADING OFF TO LONDON on 12 October 1981 to meet up with other officers joining his next ship, the *MV Devon City* in Baltimore, USA, Michael was acutely aware that Reardon Smith had in their infinite wisdom sent him everyone's tickets. His mission, which he had no choice but to accept, was to rendezvous with the rest of the party in Terminal 3 at 1 pm. As he always did, Michael hired a car to get him to the airport, but hadn't allowed enough time for any road delays. It was, of course, sod's law that the day he had to be on time, the M1 was backed up for miles. By the time he arrived an hour after he should have, the tension was palpable in the air around the other officers and their wives. Reassured that they wouldn't miss their flights, they all relaxed and introductions were made. Joining their husbands on this trip were the radio officer's and the electrician's wives. Michael liked that straight away, as having wives on board often meant that there were good social opportunities.

Arriving late in the evening, they stayed at The Lord Baltimore Hotel, which Michael recalls served the most delicious French onion soup. Even now when he thinks of it, he begins to salivate as he remembers the crunch of the croutons and the melting thick layer of cheese that clung to his teeth as he ate. As Baltimore has a very nice marine area, the evening was complete after a wander around in the fresh air. The following day, and not unusually, the ship's agent arrived to tell them that the *Devon City* hadn't yet arrived but was due in the next day. Once again, Michael and his colleagues were able to be tourists and enjoy the luxury of their swish hotel.

A day or so later Michael arrived at the port to see that the *Devon City* had already started loading. Whilst he can't remember what was going into the holds, he clearly recalls the dozen or more containers which were being loaded on deck. Though none of the ships in the Reardon Smith fleet were container carriers, on occasion they would lash the big and bulky boxes to the deck, as it created a bit of extra income—as it did on this particular voyage. Weighing over 20 to 30 tons, it was imperative that the lashings were strong and numerous, so that when the ship pitched and rolled, they wouldn't move. The containers were secured with strong steel wire cables about one inch thick and tightened up with bottle screws for extra security. Each container was tightly held with at least six lashings at each end. Twelve in all would be more than enough. So they thought!

As they got set to depart, they were advised that the weather beyond the mouth of the River Delaware was bad. The crew double checked that all the lashings were secure and battened down the hatches ready to meet what Neptune had in store for them. Dropping off just inside the river mouth, the river pilot

WATCH OUT!

Heavy weather

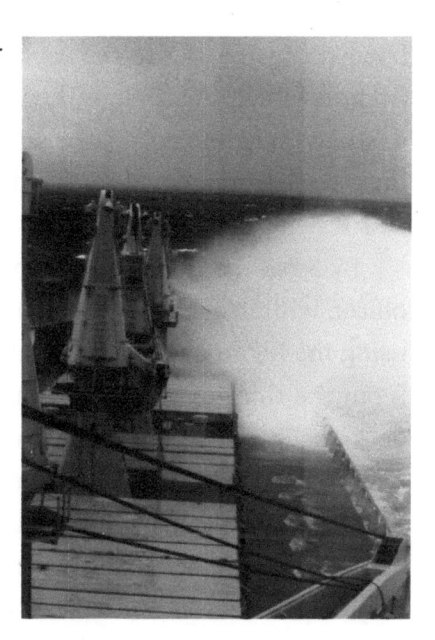

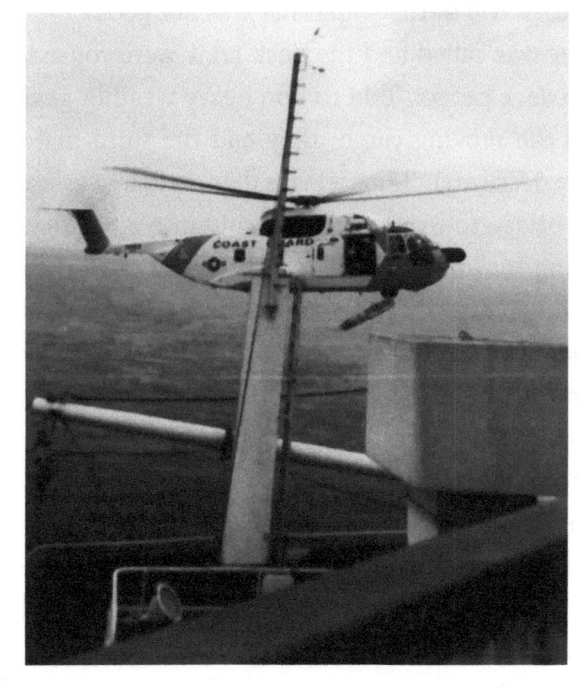

US Coast Guard airlifting injured chief officer from MV Devon City

handed control over to the captain to take his ship out into the Atlantic Ocean. As soon as they left the lee of the land, at about 4 pm, the ship immediately began to roll and pitch, and the deeper into the Atlantic they went towards South Africa, the worse the ship's swing and sway became.

By 8 pm the chief officer handed over the watch to the third officer, with instructions to monitor the safety of the deck cargo using the high-power searchlights fitted to each bridge wing. By 9 pm the third mate began to hear creaks and groans from the decks below, but the searchlights didn't show anything amiss. Making his usual nightly appearance on the bridge at 9.30 pm, the captain was told by the third mate about the noises from the deck cargo. The searchlights were shone upon the decks again, only this time it was noticed that the four forwardmost containers were moving with each roll of the ship. That was not good!

The chief officer was called and the deck crew were roused, along with the two deck cadets. Told to don heavy weather gear and make towards the moving cargo, they and the third mate went to resecure the deck cargo. Michael was then woken to assist the captain on the bridge to manoeuvre the ship into a position to reduce the rolling motions, whilst the chief officer worked with the cadets and one of the crew, and the third mate worked with the rest of them. As the waves crashed onto the decks, the containers were washed onto the hatch coamings and back into the ship's side rails. It was imperative they were tied down soon or they would end up crashing through the rails and going overboard into the maelstrom below.

Because of the immense danger the containers presented, the chief officer told the cadets not to stand between them and the ship's hatch coamings because of the risk of getting trapped.

To bring home his point he deliberately moved into the position that the cadets were told to avoid. Suddenly, a huge wave swept a 30-ton container across the deck and crushed the chief officer. His scream was heard above the howling wind and crashing seas.

Realising what had happened, the third mate radioed the bridge to advise of the serious injury his friend had suffered. When the container started moving back towards the rails, the cadets and crew member pulled the injured officer out of harm's way and let him lay on the deck. Crushed, bloodied and unconscious. An immediate medical evacuation by helicopter was radioed through to the US Coast Guard, whilst the chief steward and mess crew ran to rescue the injured man to try to get him to the safety of the accommodation. The containers were still crashing around the decks, but they were no longer the priority. Sprung into action, the coastguard ordered the captain to turn the ship around and head back to the shelter of the river so as to reduce the distance the helicopter had to travel, as the ship was now nearly 90 miles from the coast.

At close to midnight, and with tremendous efforts, the crew finally managed to duck and weave their way around the containers to carry the laden stretcher back to shelter. Then with the ship travelling in the opposite direction to the whipping wind and savage seas, the rolling and pitching lessened, allowing the third officer and the remaining crew to at long last reharness the rogue containers.

An hour later the coastguard helicopter arrived, but with nowhere for them to land, they had to lower a winchman to stretcher the injured man up into the aircraft's belly. The wind had other ideas and blew too severely to allow the winchline to be safely lowered to the deck.[7] The pilot tried many times to position his craft over the stricken vessel, but the wind was just too strong and it couldn't be done. There was no choice but to wait for them to reach the river and the ship to steady so a safe platform for the line to be lowered onto could be created. The lee of the land would reduce the apparent wind force and allow the helicopter to manoeuvre better. But that was a few hours away.

Morphine was administered to the poor injured man, but the pain was so severe it only took the edge off. He was crushed from the waist down and the soles of his rubber sea boots were split in half end to end. Despite the best efforts of the crew to get the stretcher inside the accommodation, the pain this caused was too great, and they ended up with him under the decks above but just outside the doors into the accommodation. He was smothered in blankets and given morphine shots regularly, but that was the best that could be done for him. How he survived, to this day Michael just doesn't know.

Once into the lee of the land, the helicopter returned and the poor fellow was whisked away to hospital. With the ship safely berthed, the cargo lashings were checked and an investigation started. It was soon found that the bottle screws were not of an approved make and had been purchased on the cheap by the stevedores in Baltimore. Their cheating ways were ultimately the cause of the problem. The stevedore company went on to face charges from the US authorities, though Michael was never told of the outcome.

---

[7] Helicopters create an enormous amount of static electricity, such that when they lower a line to a ship, the line has to be 'earthed' in the sea before it can be moved onto the ship.

Poor M, the injured chief officer, spent two years in hospital in America before he was well enough to be flown back to the UK. How he fared and what the long-term consequences to his health were, Michael never found out either. Sadly, he couldn't claim compensation from Reardon Smith, as, though he was demonstrating what *not* to do to the cadets, he was ultimately guilty of doing a seriously stupid thing.

Minus one officer down, the ship left port in better weather than they'd had previously, and it was agreed that Michael would take over much of the chief officer's work, whilst the third officer would take over some of his work, until such a time as a replacement chief officer could be flown out to join them.

As well as keeping the four to eight watch, it was Michael's job to get the deck crew organised and set to making repairs or doing planned maintenance to the hatches, winches, cranes or whatever else needed attention. One of the jobs he got them to do was to replace the lifting cable on one of the five cranes on deck, which involved reeling out the old cable under power and hauling the thick cable along the deck to lay it out. Next the ponder ball and hook had to be disengaged from the cable. The hook on its own weighed about 50 kg, and the ponder ball probably 200 kg, so they had to be secured in a position that would allow them to be affixed to the new cable once that cable had been fixed inside the crane. With the cable being somewhere around 100 metres long and at about 60 millimetres in diameter, it was extremely heavy.

Inside the crane, the end of the old cable was released from the heavy gauge wire clamps that held it to the drum. The cable was then tied to a heavy rope before being allowed to go through the blocks that fed the cable to the end of the jib and down onto the deck. The point of attaching the rope was so that it could be fastened to the drum end of the replacement cable and the power of the crane could slowly haul the new cable inside the crane housing and onto the drum, where it was clamped into place. Once the cable was very securely bolted in the clamps, the cable could then be hauled into its place around the drum using the power of the crane. When most of the cable was inside the crane, it was then possible to bolt the ponder ball to the remaining length of cable and lastly to secure the crane hook. This complete process took around eight hours by six crew members. With recent events fresh in their minds, the whole crew made sure that all fixtures and fittings were not only fit for purpose, but purposeful in their fit.

In addition to the deck work Michael had to oversee was the less interesting task of maintaining the records of crew working hours, overtime, sick days and days off. Ship paperwork was something that took him straight back to his early days of feeling sick when leaving port! UGH! Fortunately, he got on well with the electrician's wife, Sue, who helped with typing up the records and any other paperwork that was required.

Going to sea as an officer's wife, seeing exotic places and enjoying the freedom of the ship may sound glamorous, but the reality can be far from it. Sue's husband worked the daily eight till five shift, which meant she was free to do what she wanted for the majority of the day. Sunbathing all day every day may sound fantastic, but it soon gets boring, and doing paperwork for Michael and some of the other officers doesn't totally fill each day either. The passage from the USA to Cape Town, the next port of call, was quite boring for her, so she would often join whoever was on watch to learn how to steer the ship or have a chat, but even that has its limits. Because of Sue's help, Michael found that he got on very well with her and her husband, and they would often socialise together. The radio officer's wife also suffered from boredom, so after 14 days at sea, everyone, but especially the two ladies, was glad to arrive in Cape Town.

A highlight for Michael in Cape Town was going to the top of Table Mountain with some other officers and the on-board wives, but other than that he doesn't remember very much. Back on board the ship, they coast-hopped around South Africa, eventually arriving in Durban, where the replacement chief officer joined them. Though Michael and the third mate had been working short-handed, they were paid their normal salary plus half of the salary of the person they were covering for—so Michael not only got his own earnings, but half of the chief officer's pay too. Nevertheless, he was glad to have the new chief officer on board.

With a little less responsibility, he was able to let his hair down more, so when they got to Durban he made the most of going into town with Sue and her husband, as well as going to the funfair located on the beach front, where they all had such a good time one might have thought they were just big kids. Of course, after the trauma at the beginning of the voyage, it is not surprising they needed to let off some steam.

Wanting to see some of South Africa away from the coast, Michael, another officer and the two wives decided to hire a car one day and go exploring. With no plan of where to go, they just took one of the main roads out of Durban and went where the road took them. Stopping at a roadside restaurant for some lunch, Michael was disappointed their French onion soup wasn't a match compared to the bowl he'd had in Baltimore.

Not wanting to stay on the main highway, they turned off onto a dirt road. Thinking nothing of it, they continued on.

Apartheid was still in place and had they thought about it a little more they may have doubled back, but happy to be having an adventure they continued along the almost jungle track, until going through a large native village, they were spooked by the surprised looks from its inhabitants and realised that there were no other white people around. Once clear of the village, they stopped and collectively agreed that it wasn't safe to continue and turned the car around, hoping and praying that they wouldn't get a puncture or break down as they trundled back through the village. This time, the looks felt much more hostile, so until they got back to where the tarmac began, they avoided any direct eye contact with any of the villagers. Though they'd half expected the locals to chase after them, they were relieved when all they did was stare. Nevertheless, they high-tailed it back to the city and safety. Returning to the ship at about eight that evening, their realisation of what had happened and how close they were to getting themselves into a dangerous situation hit them. They learnt a big lesson that day and decided to stay away from black, and isolated, areas of Durban, choosing instead to only go to recognised white shops and bars.

From Durban the ship sailed to the East Coast, USA, bound for Newhaven in Long Island—the cargo of coal they had, destined for discharge back in South Africa. By the time they reached Durban the second time, the wives had been on board for around four months and were coming to the realisation that life at sea, with nothing much to do, was far from glamorous.

Michael paid off in Durban. Despite the awfulness of what had happened in Baltimore at the beginning of the voyage, Michael had had a fine trip. Because of his fondness for Sue and friendship with her husband, they stayed in touch, even after he'd returned home.

Chapter 13

Love on Land and Sea

BACK HOME IN HIS OWN HOUSE, Michael once again decided that he wanted to change his car. Driving his Vauxhall VX4/90 had made him realise how much he liked large cars, so he part exchanged it for a sumptuous, nearly new Chrysler 2 litre in metallic green.

After two and half months enjoying his new home, Michael got the call to join his next ship. The *MV Welsh City*. Sound familiar? It was the largest ship in the fleet, and though it was carrying the same name as Michael's horrible first ship, it was in fact a recent newbuild. This *Welsh City* was a 70,000 deadweight bulk carrier. She had no cranes, but seven holds, and was around 750 feet long.

Joining on his own, he didn't know who was on board so had a very pleasant surprise to find that his good friend, RS, was the captain. RS had heard the rumours going around the fleet that Michael was gay, but he also knew he'd had girlfriends. Whenever

Michael had spare time, which wasn't often, RS would invite him to his cabin for a beer and a chat, and it didn't take long to get the conversation around to his sexuality.

With no intentions of lying to him, Michael openly admitted to being bisexual. At which point, despite him having a wife and two boys back home, RS admitted he was bi-curious. He ventured further that he was attracted to Michael and had been for some time. As you can imagine, Michael was flattered.

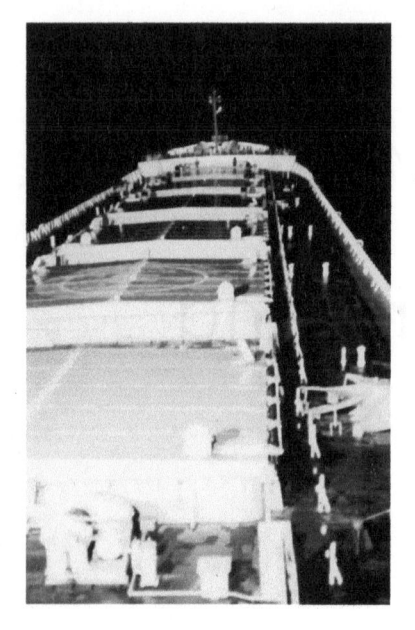

The new MV Welsh City

Michael kept the 12 to four watch, and initially RS would wander up to the bridge just after midnight to be with him. Things progressed quickly, and soon Michael was spending his 'sleeping hours' from 6 pm to midnight in RS's bunk with him. As neither of them could afford to get caught, it was a very difficult—albeit thrilling—situation, and a secret they managed to keep until the ship arrived in Baltimore, USA, where RS's voyage terminated.

Michael went from one inexplicably exciting scenario to one which left him feeling somewhat irked. RS's replacement was none other than that twat! Captain JL! Michael really wasn't happy with this turn of events, as he thought he would start his stupid rationing of the soap and toilet paper again. Happily, he was wrong. Captain JL had mellowed. He had become a real person, and a very nice one at that. Despite the problems they'd had on the previous ship, JL and Michael became good friends who got on really well together. He still had some strange ideas about life, but that was fine with Michael—he didn't have to agree with him. They sailed some interesting routes, including a trip through the Indonesian islands, running past the island of Halmahera in what was largely uncharted waters for a ship of its size. Michael eventually paid off in Singapore after almost seven months on board, flying home on 20 December 1982.

Despite having done such a long trip, his leave was relatively short, as he was due to attend college to take his Master's (captain) exams. As he still had his comfy Chrysler car, his journey to Plymouth was a delight, as was his new accommodation—

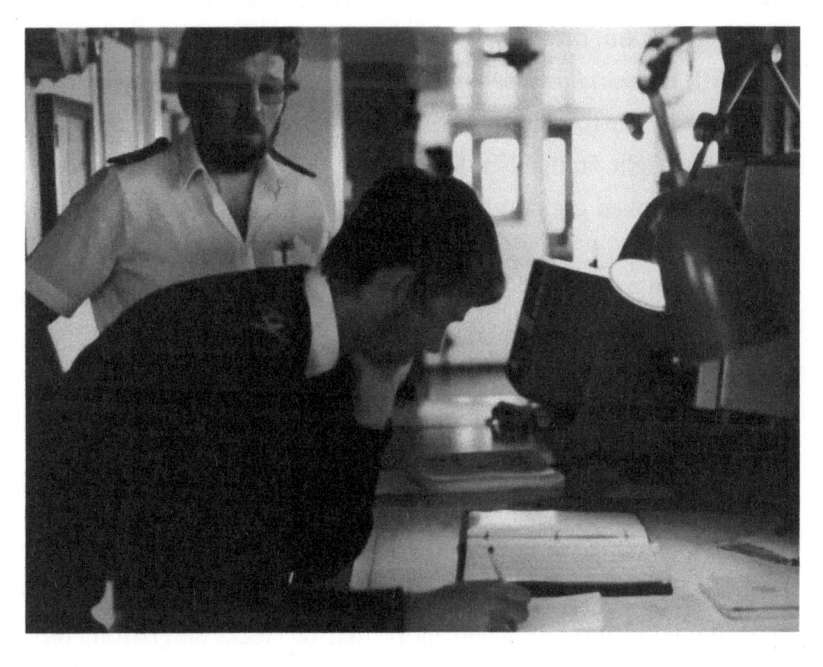

Me as 2nd officer

The Argyle Hotel—where he'd agreed to stay for the duration of his module. The hotel had an arrangement with the college, whereby they offered reduced charges for officers taking courses.

He was joined at the hotel by three or four other officers from other shipping companies: some doing their Master's certificates and others doing their first mate's qualification. Michael particularly got on well with those doing the latter, knocking around together at weekends if they didn't go home.

Having kept in touch with Sue and her husband who were back home in Bristol, Michael learnt that they were sadly getting divorced, but since they had got on so well on board the *Devon City*, Michael decided to stay in touch with Sue. So his weekends were always full, studying and hanging out with his fellow officers, staying with RS who was also on leave—and his family at their house in Devon, or going to Bristol to see Sue.

With his social life becoming much more exciting, he realised he needed a car to match, so out went the big comfy beast and in came the bright orange Fiat Mirafiori 2000TC. It was fast, sounded good and looked good, which made Michael feel good. But it was thirsty!

When RS joined his next ship, it gave Michael more time to visit Sue in Bristol. Their friendship had turned to romance, and it wasn't long before he was spending most of his weekends with her in her new house in a nice area of the city, which suited Michael as it was conveniently close to the M32 and easy for him to get to and from Plymouth.

With romance in the air, Michael found it hard to concentrate on his studies. As he had a desire to run his own business he started buying and selling jewellery, marine clocks and barometers, for which he had a ready market within the college and the other guests at the hotel. Doing well, he then branched out and purchased some TV stands which, surprisingly, he soon sold. He liked the idea of having a retail business, but being at college for a reason, he had to try to do his coursework.

As well as seamanship and navigation, the course included, amongst other subjects, engineering, law and meteorology. Michael found the latter two quite enjoyable but simply couldn't stand engineering—that was not what he'd signed up for! As captain, though, you are required to have a working knowledge of engines and engineering, whilst the opposite was not true—as chief engineer you aren't required to learn navigation!

He still had the weekends to party though, and remembers one in particular when out in his sporty car he was stopped by the police. He was obviously going too fast. Luckily he got away with just a caution. There were two other chaps in the hotel with sporty cars, and together the three of them often went out to Dartmoor to have a 'wild drive'. Michael had to be economical with the use of his car though as, despite being on full pay, expenses were high, as he had to pay the course fees himself, and the hotel, though subsidised, was not cheap. There was one occasion when he was eligible for government benefits, as his outgoings were more than his income, even though at the time, 1982/83, he was earning around £11,000 per year, which was really good money.

Despite his best efforts, Michael could not grasp engineering. It just wasn't him. Selling clocks, barometers and other things was though, and it gave him so much more pleasure than learning how engines and generators worked. At the start of the course, six months seemed a long time, but as the exams got closer, he knew that engineering was going to let him down. And though he studied hard at all subjects in the weeks before the exams, it wasn't enough. He failed engineering as he supposed he would. That meant no promotion to chief officer, but the company would allow him to resit the failed exam after another voyage.

Chapter 14

XXY

AS MICHAEL HADN'T HAD his full leave following his seven-month trip on the *Welsh City*, his leave was extended following his exams. In November 1983, once again deserting the grey skies of the East Midlands, he found himself in the warmth of Tampa, Florida, joining the *MV Port Alberni City* again. It would be his third trip on the ship—once as cadet and twice as second officer.

Their cargo this time was timber, stowed on top of the hatch lids on deck. As he was walking across the top of this cargo one day, Michael lost his footing and fell about eight feet to the deck below. Badly shaken but nothing broken, he put it down to experience and continued with his duties as normal.

Within a few weeks of his fall he noticed that he was beginning to develop breasts. Something very strange was going on. Not being able to tell anyone, he couldn't go without a shirt when on watch, as he needed to hide his growing mammaries. As the ship headed from the Indian Ocean, down the Malacca Straits and into

Singapore for fuel and stores, Michael's chest increased to a good 'B' size. Then he found a lump in the right breast. Unsure what to do, he eventually confided in the captain.

It was agreed that he would go to the hospital in Singapore as soon as they dropped anchor, to get his lump checked out. In 1983/84 Singapore was nowhere near the city it now is, and at the time Michael was whisked away by launch and taxi for the medical review, it had just one hospital.

The doctor confirmed Michael had pronounced gynaecomastia[8] and that he had a large lump, measuring about four inches by one inch, in his right breast. He was given a letter for the captain stating that he needed surgery to remove the lump and for tests to be carried out.

Reardon Smith were informed and suggested Michael had the surgery in Singapore. As it was major surgery, he declined their offer and insisted on being repatriated back to the UK in order to be seen by his GP and local hospital. He flew home with all sorts of thoughts racing through his head on the 31 January 1984.

By this time Sue had moved from Bristol and was living in Michael's house, and they were planning their wedding for his next leave. Before he'd joined his last ship, he'd rented a small shop in Wellingborough, which Sue was going to run, selling jewellery, unusual gifts, clocks and the like. He named it Embersea Gifts—playing on his initials: M ber C, which he thought was cool. Some people, though, thought it was Embassy, the cigarette brand, and wanted to know what gifts they could get in exchange for the tokens they had saved up!

---

8 Gynaecomastia is a common condition that causes boys' and men's breasts to swell and become larger than normal.

Whilst he was on the *Port Alberni City*, Sue ran the shop, and although they were very exclusive, they soon realised, when their 1983/84 Christmas sales weren't very promising, that it wasn't the kind of stuff that the people of Wellingborough wanted—unlike another local gift shop that sold tat, which had people queuing out of the door.

Disturbingly, Sue was the target of a gang of youths who came into the shop one day, and while some of them kept her attention, others were stealing what they could put into their pockets. When Michael arrived home at the end of January, they had so much to catch up on, what with the shop and his new chest. Like him, Sue was very concerned at the large lump he had. To make his chest more comfortable, Michael wore tight boob tubes which had the added advantage of flattening his chest, making him feel much less embarrassed in public.

Within a couple of days of being back, he had been seen by his GP and referred to a consultant at Kettering General Hospital. That time is a bit of a blur for Michael, and whilst he knows he must have had X-rays and scans, what he remembers most were all the blood tests he had every day for about a week. The doctors were trying to establish why he had developed such becoming boobs!

He was eventually diagnosed with Klinefelter's Syndrome. A chromosome disorder that only affects men and means he has an extra female chromosome—47, XXY. Michael was born half male, half female, which is also known as 'intersex'.

Michael was introduced to the surgeon who would be carrying out the lump removal: a famous local surgeon who had been knighted, who saw him two or three times at his private clinic in the Headlands in Kettering. On the last occasion, Michael was advised that the surgeon was going to operate the coming Tuesday. It was the Friday before and he wanted to know by Monday—did Michael want a mastectomy and to stay male, or did he want a lumpectomy and a full sex change? Shockingly, he had very little time to make up his mind. "WOW!" thought Michael. "A life-changing decision and only two days to decide!"

He went back home to break the news to Sue. Neither of them could quite grasp the enormity of the question Michael had been asked. They agonised all weekend as to what to do. Sue wanted the best for Michael, but wasn't quite sure how to handle him having a sex change. After further thought, she told him that if he did have a full sex change, she would want him to dress male, as she didn't want to be seen with him as a woman.

In the end they agreed that Michael would have the mastectomy. After all, he'd never considered himself to be female, despite his liking for feminine things. He'd also just left a very macho job, where he considered himself to be male, and was looking forward to becoming Sue's husband.

So in mid February 1984, Michael had a mastectomy. In hindsight, it was a mistake, but he wasn't to know that.

Part Three

Charting New Seas

Chapter 15

On the Road

FOLLOWING HIS OPERATION, Michael remained an in-patient for 10 days. His chest was heavily bandaged so he couldn't see what had been done. He noticed, however, that he had problems using his right arm, as the diagonal cut from his right underarm, across his nipple and towards his middle had damaged his arm muscles.

Following his discharge, he was seen by the surgeon and the consultant on several occasions. The surgeon was quite pleased that he had managed to keep his nipple, albeit with a scar through it; though, worryingly, he never mentioned the damage to his arm muscles.

To promote his masculinity, Michael was put on testosterone tablets, which he was told would be for the rest of his life. Reardon Smith gave him six months' sick leave on full pay then three months on half pay. In this time he had regular visits to his local physio department to rebuild his arm muscles.

Once his medical leave had completed, he was told to attend a Merchant Navy medical board examination in London to check if he was fit for return to a sea-going job. His general fitness was good and he had no problems. However, as he was now on hormone therapy, the examiner declared him medically unfit, as it was deemed impossible to guarantee the supply of testosterone at some of the lesser developed countries he would visit around the world. So, in September 1984, 12 years and one day after embarking on his marine career, he was declared medically unfit and discharged from the Merchant Navy.

Whilst this was unexpected, Michael was inwardly pleased, as it meant he could be Sue's husband and be with her each day. They had got married in May 1984 at Wellingborough Registry Office, followed by a small reception at a local hotel and then a short honeymoon just outside Brighton. As money was tight, they could not afford a massive reception or honeymoon, but it didn't matter—they were together and they were happy.

Being medically discharged gave Michael a medical pension, which, whilst not a fortune, helped him enormously. The pension was index linked and guaranteed until he was 55, after which he would get the Reardon Smith private retirement pension.

During one of his shore leaves whilst he was second officer, he had bought himself an HGV driving course and exam, which he passed first time. This qualified him as an HGV Class 3 driver, able to drive twin-axle trucks up to 16 tons laden weight, or to drive a twin-axle truck with a close-coupled twin-axle trailer of combined weight of 32 tons.

So from transporting thousands of tonnes of cargo around the world, he now had a new job transporting 16 tons of cargo by road. One of his first road haulage trips was an agency job working for BRS Haulage, delivering perishable goods to shops in and around Birmingham. He remembers this well, as he had found the twin gearbox difficult to use because it had a normal set of four gears like a car, then a hydraulic 'gate' to push the gearstick through to another set of four gears sitting at the side of the first one. Reverse was a real problem for him, and he ended up jamming himself against the cab door and kicking the gearstick into reverse, as it was too stiff to do it by hand. As he was delivering to narrow side entrances to shops and supermarkets, he had to use reverse gear several times and now wonders what people must have thought seeing him wedged against the driver's door and kicking the gear lever.

Another agency job Michael had was delivering building materials for a well-known builders' merchants. He had a full load on a flatbed truck that was nearly brand new and ran into difficulties approaching Brackley in Northamptonshire whilst going up the gentle hill to reach the town. He doesn't know how he did it, but he somehow managed to burn the clutch out! He was about half a mile from the town and totally blocking his lane of traffic.

As mobile phones were not in existence, Michael had to walk into Brackley and phone the depot manager to let him know he had broken down. He was not best pleased. They arranged for a tow truck to fetch him and take him to a repair yard back in Northampton. They had also delivered an empty replacement truck for the cargo to be trans-shipped onto, and he then had to go back to the building site in Brackley to deliver his load.

On arrival at the building site the site foreman advised him to drive off the tarmac road and onto the mud to get to the area where they would unload the truck. Uh oh! Another mistake! Whilst the earth looked solid, Michael had no problem reversing the truck to where they had indicated, but he failed to factor in that the 16 tons pressing down on the rear tyres would cause them to sink in the mud—which, of course, they did.

With the truck empty, Michael no longer had the grip in the rear wheels to gain traction to get out of the large ruts he had scoured into the earth. Oh shit! Now what? he thought. He ended up being half dragged out of the mud by the builder's forklift, which lifted one side of the back end and gave him slight traction to get out of the muddy area. When he eventually got back to the depot in Northampton—some three to four hours later than expected—he was told they no longer wanted his services. Not only had he damaged a nearly new truck, but he'd arrived back so late that the planned next delivery had to be cancelled and rescheduled for the next day—with a driver who knew what they were doing!

As Michael had been driving through an agency, it didn't affect him work-wise, and he was soon paired up with another transport company. This time it was with a national parcel company that had a depot in Earls Barton. He had to take a fully laden truck to Devizes and swap it for an empty truck for the return journey. This suited Michael much better. He got on well with the company he was hired out to, and his work with them was extended from one day to several weeks. After doing this run in the daytime for several days, he was asked to switch over to doing the night shift—starting at midnight and finishing around 8 or 9 am. Having worked silly hours whilst he was at sea, these hours didn't bother him; in fact, he preferred it, as there was nowhere near the amount of traffic on the roads.

Not long after starting the night shift, Michael was told that he would now be driving a wagon and drag—a lorry with a close-coupled trailer, as opposed to an articulated truck. Though you needed a Class 1 to drive an 'artic', the wagon and drag was actually harder to drive, as you cannot reverse a close-coupled trailer, because there are two pivot points: one being the towing hitch and the other the leading axle of the trailer. So whenever you stopped anywhere, you had to make sure you could drive out forwards, as there was no going back. Michael liked the wagon and drag—not just because it was extra money, but he actually enjoyed the responsibility of driving such a large awkward load.

His work with this firm ended after a few months and he was offered a contract to drive 16 tons of processed chickens to freezer storage units up and down the country. It was long-distance truck driving for a chicken processing plant in Brackley—but no mud this time. He had to start at 4 am each morning with a preloaded Volvo truck taking the loads to Newcastle, Durham, Brighton and other distant places. There was a pallet truck in the back, and he had to reverse onto a loading bay and then manouevre each stack of pallets from the back of the truck and onto the loading dock. Though it was cold in the back of the freezer truck, he soon worked up a sweat moving the pallets around.

Michael got on well with the chicken firm's transport manager, and it wasn't long before he was offered a permanent contract, working for them direct and cutting the agency out. Under the agency's contract, this arrangement was not allowed without some financial penalty to the firm making the offer. But that was their problem, not Michael's. So he accepted the position and became a chicken company employee.

In the Merchant Navy, Michael's final salary was £11,000 a year, so he was really happy landing this driving job, as he was on the same amount of £11,000, though not, sadly, tax free. After working on the long-distance work for a few weeks, he was called into the manager's office and asked if he wanted to go on their smaller 7.5-ton, multi-drop delivery trucks. For this he got a pay rise, had to wear a company tie and got his own permanent round. Naturally, he accepted, and was soon delivering to about 20 fried chicken outlets in and around London.

To beat the traffic as much as possible, he had to be at his first city drop-off by 6 am each day, so again he was starting at 4 am. Though these were smaller trucks, the job was more demanding, as he had to deliver to each outlet, often in narrow or crowded streets, and constantly be on the lookout for traffic wardens who tried to enforce the 'no loading' rules in many of the places he had to deliver to.

Despite all of this, he got on very well, until one day, on returning to the depot, the transport manager told him he had some bad news for him. This threw Michael, as his immediate thought was that something had happened to Sue. Instead, he was told that his car had been damaged on the road outside their offices. What had happened was that a truck had been parked behind his car, which wasn't a problem, but another driver had unhitched an artic trailer in front of his car and had forgotten to set the trailer brake. The gentle incline in the road was enough to set the trailer moving backwards into his bonnet and physically push his car onto the truck behind. So his Lada Riva—yes, you read that right; he had a Lada—was now about 12 inches shorter, with the front end quite mangled and the rear end compressed.

Michael was given the manager's car to get home in and was told they would sort out the insurance claim in the morning. When he returned for work the next day, the fitters had bent the front wings into a position that allowed Michael to drive it home. They didn't stick to their promise though and never put in the insurance claim, so Michael ended up leaving the company and issuing proceedings against them. His car was fixed at their expense and all his legal fees were paid.

Chapter 16

Hormonal Horrors

FROM THE DAY OF MICHAEL'S discharge from the Merchant Navy, he began taking testosterone tablets twice a day. Initially these worked well, but as his testosterone levels improved, he found he was becoming more and more irritable and aggressive. Constant arguing with Sue and his parents, coupled with early road-rage, were worrying signs.

Having recently moved from their house in Wellingborough to a larger one in a pleasant cul-de-sac in the village of Earls Barton, Michael and Sue were still in the process of getting to know their neighbours. They got on well with one set, whilst the other was a single lady in her later years whom they rarely saw. The house opposite was occupied by a retired police superintendent who rumour had it was intolerant to others. About 12 months after moving in, this particular neighbour got the builders in to add a new rear extension to his property.

The builders, seemingly oblivious to the other residents, started work at six every morning and thought nothing of making all sorts of loud noises. Michael put up with the disturbance for three or four days but then snapped. As far as he was aware the law allows noise from 7 am, so in his frustration he made an anonymous phone call to the builders' firm stating that he was going to sue them for breach of the peace.

Of course his neighbour soon heard about this and somehow knew straight away that it was Michael who had made the call. His retaliation was swift. He encouraged the builders to make as much noise as they could, tried to prevent Michael's father from parking his car outside his son's house and attempted to get the police to stop Michael from parking anywhere other than on his own drive. Clearly the former police superintendent also had a lot of testosterone flying around, and Michael feels sure that had this situation occurred now, whilst he is on oestrogen, not testosterone, it would all have been handled in a much calmer, more appropriate manner. Being on testosterone made him nasty.

The reality of this really hit home on another occasion, when visiting a gay bar with friends in Northampton, he refused to queue at the bar to be served. Instead he elbowed his way through the crowd and upon reaching the bar demanded to be served. Realisation struck him. His behaviour was both rude and aggressive, and it was all down to testosterone. At some point Michael's medication was changed from tablets to testosterone injections (Sustanon) in his buttocks every two weeks. It was literally a fortnightly pain in the bum! Although the method of receiving the hormone had changed, the effects did not. Two further incidents occurred, which Michael puts down to the negative side effects of his hormone therapy.

On one occasion, whilst returning his lorry to the chicken processing yard, he got into a road-rage situation with a car towing a caravan. The car driver nearly took his wing mirror off, their vehicles got so close. One might imagine the air was very blue. Another time, Michael had a run-in with another lorry driver in London, who caused him to stop his truck and then proceeded towards him, his intentions clear: he was looking for a fight. Though Michael was aggressive, he wasn't stupid, and seeing that this opponent was twice his size, he locked his cab doors and reversed out of the situation. How trans men cope with taking testosterone nowadays Michael cannot understand; it still has the same side effects.

After being on testosterone for six or seven years, Michael chose, against his doctor's advice, to stop taking it. His GP was not happy and kept insisting that Michael take the male hormone, because, well, he *was* male. He simply didn't seem to grasp that Michael wasn't a full-bloodied male, but half male and half female. By taking the testosterone Michael would only be increasing his masculinity because that was what the medics thought he should do. But Michael knew differently. He knew that being male and being aggressive were not the real him. He wanted to explore his feminine side and to try taking oestrogen.

In 1993, about a year after stopping the testosterone, Michael asked his doctor to prescribe him oestrogen. He was once again told that he was male, and so it was not possible. How could he make his doctor accept and understand that he wasn't? Every time he saw him, he reiterated his request. After much cajoling, Michael's doctor finally agreed to a three-month trial. Asked how he was feeling at the end of the three months, Michael's answer couldn't have been clearer: "Fantastic!" he exclaimed. Somewhat baffled, his doctor could not see how that could be. Michael was, in his expert medical opinion, a man. How could Michael possibly make him understand that he wasn't?

HORMONAL HORRORS

During this time, Michael had set up his new business adventure: Marine Chart Services. One Saturday in April 1993, whilst teaching navigation skills to a bunch of yachtsmen at his office premises, he suddenly felt a sharp pain in his right lung. Thinking it was just wind or indigestion, he dismissed it and continued with the class until it ended at one. Driving home, he was aware that the pain on his right side was still there. Upon reaching home he mentioned it to Sue, who also dismissed it as nothing much to worry about.

That afternoon, they went to an open-air craft market at Lilford Hall and Michael began to have great difficulty walking around due to the pain. Eventually, they abandoned their plans and returned home where he succumbed to lying on the settee, as

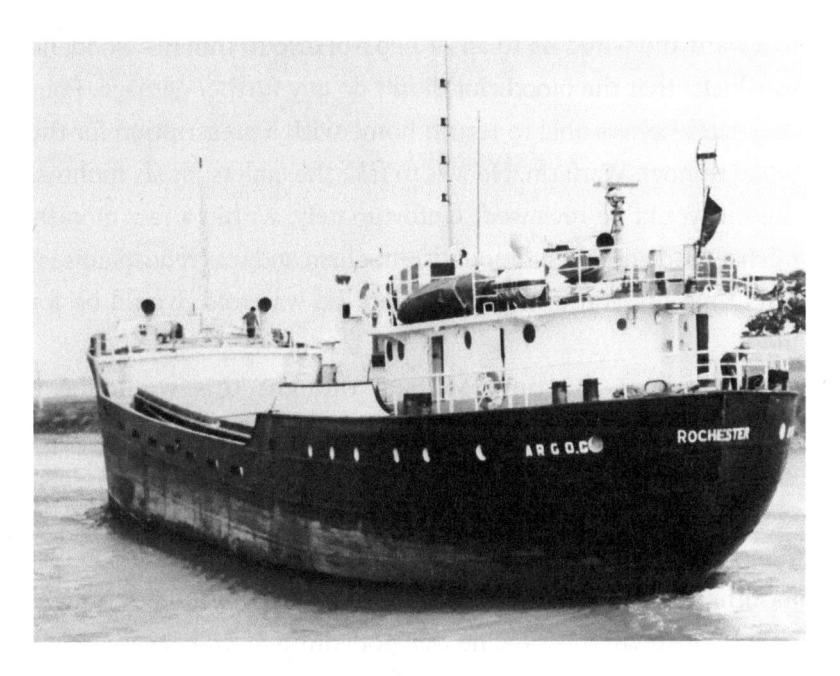

One of the first clients of Marine Chart Services

it seemed to lessen the pain. Worried that he wasn't getting better, Sue eventually called the doctor, who, upon hearing Michael's symptoms, agreed that a home visit was necessary. It was clearly urgent, as he arrived within 30 minutes, diagnosed the problem and gave Michael an injection in his backside. Sue was told to take her husband to the A&E department at Northampton General Hospital immediately. When asked what was wrong with Michael, he said that he was having a pulmonary embolism (PE)—a blood clot in the lung—a serious and life-threatening condition. To say that Michael was shocked would be an understatement.

Arriving at the hospital, Michael struggled into A&E and was soon being treated. He has not forgotten the sight of a needle being put into his wrist and, upon finding the artery, seeing the blood spurt out. Neither has he forgotten the pain it caused. Admitted to a ward and wired up to an IV heparin drip to thin his blood, he was lucky that the blood clot didn't do any further damage. Four days later he was able to return home with a prescription for the blood thinner, Warfarin. He was to take the tablets for six months, then it would be reviewed. Unfortunately, within a few months Michael had another pulmonary embolism and was rehospitalised. This time his Warfarin prescription, he was told, would be for life.

Though at the time Michael thought this would be a metaphorical pain in the butt, as he would have to attend a clinic to have the hypercoagulability—or in layman's terms, the thickness of his blood—checked once or sometimes twice a week, as thicker, stickier blood is more likely to form clots than thinner blood. Six months later Michael suffered another PE, and though he was seen in hospital, this time he was not admitted, as he was already taking the recommended treatment to stop clots from forming. The trouble was it wasn't working. It would be a long time before either Michael or the medics put two and two together and realised that it was the oestrogen that was causing the clots to form.

Despite the three PEs Michael had had, he was given another three-month trial of oestrogen a few years later. Again it made him feel really good, and yet his doctor continued to pooh-pooh this notion, as Michael was male. As he had no intention of ever going back to being the aggressive person testosterone turned him into, he continued to push for oestrogen. Alas, to no avail.

With access to a computer at work, Michael took advantage of the newly found Internet and searched the web to find an overseas source of Progynova (oestrogen) and Cyproterone (testosterone blockers). The source, The Garden Pharmacy, was located in the Pacific Islands, and to this day Michael doesn't know if the drugs were real or fake, but for him they worked. He felt better, calmer and more in control, so he continued to buy from the Internet. Of course, he still hadn't realised that oestrogen was the root cause of his blood clots. He continued to take the tablets until 2007, when following a minor operation, for which he had to pause taking Warfarin, he had a heart attack.

Chapter 17

Nude and Rude!

INITIALLY, MICHAEL FELT a sharp pain in his chest, but as he had just been given an intravenous bolus of heparin, he didn't think anything was wrong. Nothing to worry about, he thought, and carried on chatting with his mum and stepdad who were visiting him at the time. But as the pain continued to get worse, he called for a nurse. Being in a private hospital, help came very quickly, and when Michael told the nurse about the pain in his chest, she bleeped the on-call doctor immediately. He arrived within a couple of minutes and, as Michael's visitors left the room, he gave him another shot of heparin. It made no difference. The pain surged and the doctor called 999, as Michael was having a heart attack. Being a private hospital, there were no facilities to treat emergencies, so Michael was rushed to Kettering General Hospital by ambulance.

Managing somehow to get a quick phone call in to Sue to bring her up to date, when he arrived at A&E he was transferred to the 'majors' area and hooked up to monitors. Within minutes, he was being treated and having initial blood tests to check his troponin levels, which if raised would prove conclusively that he was indeed having a heart attack. Having already been sick in the ambulance, due to the fast and bumpy ride, he threw up again once he was settled. Things were not looking good. That evening, he was transferred to the assessment ward, had more blood tests and waited for the results. They came back positive. Michael had had his first coronary.

He was moved to the heart ward where he stayed for a week until being transferred to Glenfield Hospital in Leicester. Michael had been told that he would be under the care of Dr McCann, but that didn't happen, as tragically it was his daughter, Madeleine, who was abducted from the villa in Portugal. Michael's care was taken over by another heart specialist.

At Glenfield, Michael had an angiogram,[9] which revealed there was no arterial build-up or visible damage. That meant that a blood clot had travelled up to Michael's heart and caused his heart attack. He was still on oestrogen tablets, just as he was when he had the previous pulmonary emboli, and still no one put two and two together—least of all Michael.

A week later he was discharged and told to take two weeks off work to rest and recuperate. That was not easy for Michael, and going round and round in his mind were a number of 'what ifs', so for reasons that he still doesn't completely understand, he decided to get a second opinion. His private cardiologist confirmed the diagnosis and Michael accepted that he had to learn to relax.

---

9 Where a tube and camera are inserted into your artery through your wrist or groin, allowing doctors to see if there has been damage to your arteries and heart.

Two boring weeks with nothing to do were made bearable, as he was able to spend them with Sue, who having left her accountancy job to be Michael's business manager in 1999 was now running his business for him. Though part of his rehabilitation was to attend a heart attack recovery group at Kettering General Hospital, where he joined in with gentle exercises to improve his heart function, when it ended after eight weeks he was glad that he could continue his life, with Marine Chart Services as his main focus.

It wasn't long before fate disrupted his routine again. Having developed some problems with his mobility around August 2007, he went to get checked out at hospital in Northampton. Astonishingly, he was turned away, but as he was walking back to his car he collapsed in the car park. Help was quickly summoned and he was then admitted for tests and observation, eventually being transferred to Rowan Ward for monitoring. Not long afterwards, Michael found that he wasn't able to pee properly. This too was dismissed as a minor problem, but things soon grew a lot worse when Michael found he couldn't pee at all. Given a bottle by the nurses, he was told that the pressure of the fluid build-up in his bladder would cause the blockage to ease and he would eventually go. How wrong they were! After six hours of not passing urine, he was in pain, but still nothing happened. After 12 hours a doctor was called and painkillers prescribed. The medics still agreed that the blockage would eventually clear itself. After 23 hours and in immense pain, feeling that his bladder would burst out of his skin, they finally conceded and decided to insert a catheter. The relief was so overwhelming that Michael collapsed and passed out. Passing nearly three litres of fluid so quickly is apt to do that to a man! To Michael's further relief, the catheter was left in ready to be removed a couple of days later when his bladder function would be checked.

That day soon arrived, and Michael was told to keep drinking plenty of fluids to allow his bladder to fill up, which would cause him to pee. Nothing happened. Though he had been given strong painkillers to prevent any more agony, his bladder wouldn't function, and after another achingly long 23 hours he was recatheterised.—the relief once again causing him to pass out. The doctors then agreed that Michael would need to have a permanent catheter. By this time, he had been on Rowan Ward for almost four weeks and was feeling more and more down. He remembers feeling so depressed one evening that he cried all night and into the next morning. A psychiatrist was called to see him and he was put on low dose antidepressants. Eventually, six weeks after initially being turned away for a problem with his mobility, he was discharged from hospital complete with catheter and drainage bags.

Before being beset by these medical problems, Michael had been working as a lorry driver, but following the chicken-firm car-trashing incident, looked elsewhere for work. Being open to all sorts of challenges, he answered an advert for an artist's model at Nene College in Northampton.[10] During an informal interview with the head of art, he was advised that the work would be both clothed and unclothed. Being nude didn't bother Michael, so he was soon sitting down in nothing, doing nothing,—and being paid for it! His time was in much demand, and Michael wondered why other models weren't being used. When told that the art department had great difficulty finding models, he was

---

10 Now the University of Northampton.

very surprised—not least because there were around two million unemployed people at the time. Ever the entrepreneur, Michael offered to find the models if the college assured him they would employ them.

And so Mike Clarke Art Models was founded. Advertising at Job Centres in Wellingborough and Northampton, he soon had about a dozen models on his books. He hit that all too common problem of supply and demand, with too many models and not enough work. Always ready with a solution, Michael started canvassing senior schools and colleges in and around Northamptonshire, and before too long his modelling services were well known in the art world. With around 30 models on his books, working within a 50-mile radius of Northampton, business was booming.

Whilst modelling was okay, Michael's heart was not really in it. He was, he realised, all at sea without a maritime connection, so, with some professional help in August 1986, he set up Marine Chart Services. He canvassed around 1,000 shipping companies all over the UK and Europe and got just one response, which went nowhere. Then the BBC and ITV news got wind of his business and he was given a few minutes coverage by each station in their prime-time local news programmes. Still no work came in.

Sue, who was now working as an accountant with a small firm in Northampton, advised him to give up MCS and look for a proper job. Undeterred, Michael selectively canvassed individual UK shipping companies until one day he was commissioned to do some work for Sealink Ferries in Dover.

He'd also been keeping an eye on the job vacancies advertised in some motor yacht magazines, when one job, for a captain of a large multimillion pound yacht belonging to a British millionaire, caught his attention. Michael knew without a doubt that he had to have that job, so he carefully wrote out his CV and sent it in. Though he was doing a few odd jobs for Sealink at the time, he felt he could fit both jobs into his work schedule.

A few weeks later Michael got a phone call from the millionaire asking him to go to his house, which turned out to be a mansion, in Royal Tunbridge Wells to attend an informal interview. Michael clearly remembers there being a large wishing well in the massive garden and must have subliminally wished for his dream to come true. Whether it was his experience, qualifications and things he talked about in general during his interview, or the magic of the water feature, he was over the moon to be told at the end that he had got the job. And he had beaten the 42 other candidates to boot!

Flying to where it was moored in Amsterdam, at his new boss's expense, Michael's first experience of the luxury yacht entailed living on board for two weeks to assess what modifications would be required for it to safely convey his new employer and his wife to Menorca. Safety was paramount, as the owner had a false leg and walked with the aid of crutches. Working out how to make the massive Cheoy Lee motor yacht safe for an invalid to stand and steer, and get about the yacht safely, was not straightforward. Michael insisted on a steel support being fitted about 18 inches away from the helm, with the support bolted into the deck above and below to enable the owner to secure himself to it when he chose to steer. With numerous grab rails installed and modifications to the galley, dining spaces and out on deck, the total cost of all the alterations ran into many tens of thousands of pounds. But it didn't matter; they had to be done.

Ready to return in July to command the yacht out into the North Sea and around the coast to Gibraltar and eventually to

Mahon in Menorca, Michael needed crew and agreed that the owner would find some people he knew and Michael would bring one extra crewman with him that he knew. Additionally, Sue was allowed to go with Michael for part of the voyage as a free holiday. They flew into Amsterdam in a howling gale and a forecast that promised quite a few unsettled days ahead. Despite the adaptions that had been made to the yacht, Michael knew that it would be unsafe to enter the North Sea in those conditions and that they would have to wait for the wind and seas to calm down. This was not what the owner wanted to hear. Instead he was keen to reach their first stopover in the Channel Islands, for which he had a three-day window to arrive. Though Michael sympathised, it was, in his view as captain, unsafe for the vessel to leave port. However, he agreed to the yacht going down to Ijmuiden to wait for the weather to clear, so that they were nearer to getting into the North Sea when the right opportunity arose. That opportunity never came, as Michael and the owner had an argument as to who was in charge of the yacht. Michael made it clear that as the captain it was, in his opinion, unsafe to leave port. The owner retaliated by insisting that he was not going to miss his meeting in the Channel Islands, and—as he was the owner and Michael worked for him—demanded that they set out of the harbour.

Michael was caught between a rock and a hard place. Yes, he was the captain, but he was also an employee, and despite his arguments, had to do as he was instructed. Everything that could be secured was tied down or made safe and they left Ijmuiden and crossed the harbour bar and entered into the North Sea. It wasn't long before the waves were crashing over the decks and slamming into the wheelhouse and accommodation. Michael foretold this, but thinking he knew best, the owner didn't heed his warning.

With the waves battering the yacht, he finally admitted Michael was right and agreed that it was unsafe to continue. With some difficulty, Michael and the crew turned the yacht around and manoeuvred it back inside the shelter of Ijmuiden. The owner was fuming. Not only had he missed his meeting, but he had to admit he'd been wrong. Remaining in the shelter of Ijmuiden for a couple of days, the owner worked out his next move. His decision was to return to Amsterdam, where he abandoned the voyage, deciding to fly to his various meetings instead. Clearly not happy with his yacht's ability to tackle heavy seas, he also informed Michael that he was going to sell the yacht in Amsterdam and would buy a bigger and better yacht when he got to his new home in Menorca.

This news was a real blow to Michael, his wife and crew mate, as they had signed up for a six- to eight-week voyage, yet just a week into it, it was being abandoned. Michael's pay had been agreed at a day rate, which, had the voyage taken longer than estimated, would have compensated him for the extra time. That decision backfired, as he was only paid a fraction of the amount he had hoped for. The same went for the crew he had brought with him. So, somewhat disgruntled, the three of them flew back home and carried on working in their regular jobs.

Michael never heard from the owner or his wife again, although some of the products his companies produce can still be seen on supermarket shelves to this day. Michael prefers not to look!

Chapter 18

Blithe Spirit

BACK HOME ONCE AGAIN, Michael concentrated on getting more work for Marine Chart Services, selectively canvassing a few companies each week to ensure that if any work did come his way, he wouldn't be swamped by it. He also had some fairly regular work for Sealink, maintaining their folios of navigation charts and keeping them up to date. As they were folios which could be needed to get a vessel from Dover to a dry dock or repair yard, they could be required at very short notice. He also picked up a few jobs for a Dutch salvage-and-tug company to update the complete outfit of charts carried by each vessel whilst they were in port for repairs. It meant he had around 600 charts to manually update in a short period of time. No mean feat, which he admits stretched his abilities so much that he had to take on another chart corrector.

The new employee lived reasonably close to Michael and came from a well-known London chart agency, so knew the work required of him. Having converted one of his bedrooms into a drawing office, the new recruit worked there during the day, whilst Michael took over in the evenings to get the work done in the time allocated.

Despite his heavy workload, Michael continued canvassing other companies and had a pleasant surprise when one day he received a phone call from Ireland asking him to take over the maintenance of some 20 or so ships' chart outfits. The company had about three spare outfits of charts, and once he had updated one of these, it was couriered to a ship somewhere in the UK—often London or Liverpool. The process then repeated itself in steady rotation when another outdated set was returned in its place.

The amount of work now required Michael to rent offices, and he found just what he was looking for on Wellingborough High Street. Located on the first floor at the front, with a ramp access at the rear, and an area of 650 square feet in total, it also meant he needed additional staff. Turning to family first, he employed his mum as his office administrator and found a trainee chart corrector by advertising with the local Job Centre. The trainee, LR, turned out to be an excellent employee and soon became a very proficient chart corrector. To help her understand the meaning of the charted symbols and better comprehend the way a ship navigated with them, she was enrolled onto one of Michael's training courses and taught navigation, seamanship, meteorology and chartwork. Michael found that his original employee was abusing his position—regularly clocking up £60 of phone calls to his girlfriend when the boss was out of the office—so he had to let him go. He was soon replaced with another trainee, PF, who also turned out to be an excellent and trustworthy worker.

Word of his firm's success and proficiency soon spread around the shipping world and work steadily floated his way. By 1990

Michael was looking after around 100 ships. With opportunities to extend their services by visiting the ship in port around the UK, updating their charts on board, they were able to do the work within a twelve-hour window, meaning that the vessel retained her own valuable outfit of charts. To do so effectively meant Michael buying a van so that two members of his now expanded staff could travel to each ship in the vehicle to do the work. Visiting many ports—including those at Kings Lynn, Liverpool, Immingham, Southampton, Runcorn and London—the staff were required to work long hours, often as many as 18 where some of the more remote ports were concerned.

By 1992 Michael had up to eight members of staff and realised that he needed to find larger premises. It took until late 1993 to early 1994 before suitable premises were found, conveniently just around the corner in Oxford Street, but again on the first floor.

Before leaving the High Street offices, the team experienced some strange events within some rooms. On one occasion Michael's mother was making hot drinks for everyone and as she took a bottle of milk out of the countertop fridge, it flew out of her hand and hit the wall, spookily at the same height as her hand. This shouldn't be possible, as the weight of the bottle would have meant it would have hit the wall lower down. Then some cupboard doors in one of the back rooms suddenly burst open for no reason. When things started to go missing without explanation, Michael had had enough. He engaged a clairvoyant to try to find out what was causing these strange events. Arriving at 6 pm one evening, with a strong male friend, Michael asked her, "Why the 'heavy'?"

She responded, "If it's a malevolent spirit, I might have to be wrenched away from its effects, and a strong person is needed to do this!"

Settling down at one of Michael's classroom tables, which were about four feet by two feet with a heavy wooden top and metal legs—they were heavy tables—she summoned the spirits. Soon the table was tilting on two legs. Michael couldn't believe what he was seeing. There was no one else touching the table and she only had her fingertips touching the top surface, so she couldn't have made the table move in the way it was moving, and it was not possible for her knees to move it, as the gap was too great. She was in touch with a young boy who had died in that building many years before. His spirit was still roaming the building, which before being used as offices, used to be the servants' quarters of the adjacent mansion. The spirit boy was the son of the family that owned the property, who told the clairvoyant that he was just playing when these events happened and he didn't mean any harm. The mystic then looked into Michael's future for the business and predicted that he would move to a larger, glass-fronted office and that he would get the business of a large client, the contact of whom would be a bald German man.

The offices Michael moved to in 1994 were glass fronted, and later in that year he picked up lots of work from a large ship management company based in Cyprus. And his contact? A very nice German man with a bald head!

"Believe it or don't believe," Michael warns, "but I was there and saw and heard all this, and I truly believe in the supernatural now!"

Chapter 19

Luxury and Loss

WITH MARINE CHART SERVICES now well established, Michael decided to diversify the range of services on offer. He introduced chart audits where he would go to a ship anywhere in the world to inspect the charts. His main task was to see if the ship's navigator was doing his job properly and to provide a fully detailed report of his findings. It didn't take long before it became a sought-after service, leading to him picking up Esso Petroleum and several other big-name clients who also wanted this provision. In 1994 Michael marketed the idea of teaching navigation officers how to correct charts properly. Despite this being part of their duties, there is no actual formal training given, and each person learns from their predecessor. It stands to reason that if that individual was rubbish at correcting charts, their successor becomes incompetent too.

Quickly becoming another sought-after service, Michael's first teaching contract was to teach 12 seafarers at the Ukraine Maritime Academy in Odessa in the middle of winter. Booked for two consecutive training sessions of two days each, Michael was raring to go, but unfortunately was seriously delayed on the way to Heathrow Airport by an accident that blocked the motorway, resulting in him missing his flight. The contracted company were very understanding and expected him instead on the following day's flight, which he boarded without any problems.

On arrival at Odessa Airport the pilot told passengers to hold on tight as the plane came in to land. They soon found out why. The runway was in a very poor state, with potholes and God knows what, and the aircraft was brought to a rapid stop and then taxied to the terminal, bouncing and swaying because of the terrible road surface. Shaken but not stirred, Michael made his way to baggage control—only to find it didn't exist! Instead, all the bags were piled in a heap in the arrivals hall. After presenting his luggage receipt tag to a guard, he was allowed to take his items away. Then all he had to do was to part with $100 of his hard-earned cash for a 'visa' to get through airport security. The 'visa' being a stamp in his passport!

He was met at the airport by V, a senior naval officer in full uniform with tons of gold braid everywhere. Expecting a little bit of luxury, Michael was surprised when he was taken to his transport. Somehow he just wasn't expecting it to be a battered Renault 16. However, it took him and his gilded colleague to a floating hotel in the port of Odessa, where Michael then met up with the shipping company's training officer who had flown out on the flight he'd missed. KP was a very nice person with whom Michael got on well. All was well, and as Michael was the first western lecturer to ever teach at the academy, he was, except for the vaguely alarming airport transfer vehicle, treated like royalty. With a special trip arranged for him and KP to attend the ballet, Michael was delighted, especially since he'd never been to see the ballet before and because they were given the best seats in the house.

The next day Michael got a real sense of how things worked in the Ukraine. Arriving at the classroom, fully prepared to teach 12 students, he was surprised to find double that number eagerly awaiting him. Still, Michael wasn't a captain for nothing and was superb at making things work, even with only enough equipment for the original 12 students. When he realised that the academy was only allowed electricity two days a week, and the days he was teaching were not those two, he like everyone else just stayed wrapped up in his coat, scarf and gloves to fight off the extreme cold. No electricity also meant no lights, so the day ended when the night drew in at about 4 pm.

On their second night in Odessa, Michael and KP went for a drink and then on to the casino. With the average wage being about $20 a month, they were, in comparison to others, millionaires. It probably didn't go down too well when Michael went on to win $50 on the roulette table.

After two days teaching in the cold with a deficit of equipment, Michael and KP were more than pleased when the academy principal told them that the course had been a huge success. Everyone was made up with Michael's teaching and the topics taught. To celebrate, the principal insisted on taking them out to dinner that night, and when they offered to pay, they were quickly told that it was his treat and he wouldn't accept any payment from them whatsoever. The principal earned $50 a month, whereas Michael's fees were close to £1,000 per day! It is not money which maketh the man!

Getting ready to leave on their final day, V insisted they go via his office, where he invited his guests to have a farewell drink of whisky. Michael asked for a small one, as he'd be driving once he reached London. He was told just two fingers' worth in the glass, which he took to mean two horizontal fingers' worth, or about an inch in the glass. Not so! They meant two vertical fingers' worth, and a glass full to the brim! Not being a drinker at the best of times, and certainly not an imbiber of whisky, Michael was caught between swallowing the amber liquid or insulting his host. Though he'd had a full breakfast, he knew that much whisky was going to be a problem for him and might cause him problems driving, but offending V would be unacceptable. Whether it was the sub-zero temperature or something else, he doesn't know, but he managed to drive home from Heathrow—and without being stopped by the police.

The company that had engaged Michael to teach in Odessa reported back that it was a huge success and that they would be getting Michael to go there again. Word of his teaching success quickly reached the ears of other companies, and it wasn't long before he was teaching or auditing chart corrections all over the world, visiting Italy, Dubai, Singapore, Brazil, USA, Norway, Greece, the Philippines, South Korea, Belfast and many other places. When Michael set Marine Chart Services up, his competitors pooh-poohed his business idea, saying it wouldn't work, yet by 1994/95, he had become the world leader in chart maintenance procedures. He was well happy.

In 1996 the Crown Prosecution Service sought advice from the Nautical Institute, of which Michael is a member, to find a navigation expert who could work with them on a marine disaster case they were prosecuting. A ship had foundered off Padstow in Cornwall and several crew had died, yet the captain was one of the first to leave the stricken ship. The Nautical Institute had some

7,000 members from shipping companies far and wide, but that didn't matter—they chose Michael. Deemed to be the best of the best at navigation, he became an expert witness for the Crown Prosecution Service at the trial, which lasted for several days, at Exeter Crown Court. The outcome: the captain was found guilty of leaving his crew mates and sentenced to spend several years in prison.

Not long before this case, Michael's father Jim, to whom he was very close, died. At the time of his death, both his sister, Linda, and his mother, Edna, were on holidays overseas. Jim didn't like going on holiday, so Edna had gone on a cruise with a lady friend. Whilst Michael's brother, David, helped with the death certificates and sorting out the funeral, he contacted the cruise company and arranged for his mum to fly back to the UK from Miami. Needing to get home super quick, she flew home on Concorde, and though Jim sadly passed away the day before she arrived, afterwards Edna was able to find a silver lining in that dark cloud through her novel claim to fame: so proud was she to have travelled back in style on the most famous aeroplane in the world. Michael's pain at losing his dad was eased slightly by his remaining family members all being able to return for his father's funeral.

Chapter 20

Moving On–In More Ways Than One

MICHAEL'S SUCCESS IN TEACHING continued, as did his chart-auditing work. Not one to rest on his laurels though, he soon came up with a new idea to entice the shipping industry into his net with the launch of Sail with the Ship or Operational Procedures Audits.

Whilst sailing with the ship, Michael would observe the navigational and other procedures carried out. It usually required at least two days on board, so having joined the ship in one port, he would leave at the next. Like his previous ideas, this, too, soon caught on, and as Michael was the only person offering this service, his workload increased exponentially. The inspection voyages took him from the UK to Portugal, France and Germany, as well as a voyage down the coast of Brazil.

During this latter trip, the contracting company was looking to achieve the high standards required by an international petroleum company to allow that ship to carry their cargoes. Michael's report would be the 'yea or nay' say as to whether they won this prestigious contract. To 'assist' him in completing the report, the shipowner not only offered to fly Michael to Brazil first class but tried to entice him with an added four-figure 'bonus' to complete the job. Clearly a bribe, Michael, who takes great pride in the integrity of his work, politely refused both offers.

When he got to Brazil, having flown quite comfortably in economy, he joined the ship, only to find that all officers and crew were in a state of shock. They had just been held captive by Brazilian pirates and the ship ransacked. Whilst the crew were herded into a large room at gunpoint and locked in, the pirates ransacked every cabin of all money and valuables. They left leaving the crew still locked up. The traumatised captives eventually managed to smash the door down and call for help. It was so traumatic for the wife of the British chief engineer, who was travelling with her husband, that she had to be flown back to the UK.

Mindful of their mental state, given what they had just been through, Michael continued with his inspection. Examining procedures employed in navigating the ship, the state of all the safety equipment and the knowledge and proficiency shown in the lifeboat and fire drills Michael had them do were all done with empathy. After all, Michael could bring his own distressing experiences on board ship to bear, but the ship still had to be safe for all concerned. Regardless of recent events, the ship was badly run, badly designed and the crew had no idea how to use the safety equipment. They didn't pass Michael's inspection and, therefore, didn't get the contract they were chasing. It's hardly surprising that the owner wanted Michael to take a bribe to secure a very different outcome!

On what was meant to be a short three- or four-day trip for a client from Teesside in North East England down to Leixoes in Portugal turned into another rough crossing. The weather from the Bay of Biscay and down to Leixoes was so appalling that it delayed the ship's arrival off the port. Then, because it was too stormy to enter port, the ship had to stay at anchor for another few days until the weather improved. Unlike when he captained the millionaire's yacht, Michael was quite happy, as his 'day rate' was still being paid, even though he had nothing to do. When the ship finally arrived inside the harbour, he was told he would have to get a coach from Leixoes to Lisbon Airport as the airport in Leixoes was closed due to fog. Though they had no choice but to go with it, this was definitely not what the company wanted.

It sounds as though some companies have to show they have followed procedure, and this can mean that they engage a specialist like Michael to carry out safety checks. Such was the case when Michael was hired by a charity to inspect their two sail training vessels. Joining the first ship in Las Palmas, he sailed with this lovely craft for a week, cruising around the Canary Islands whilst looking at the operating procedures and general safety levels. At the end of the week, he transferred to the second ship and spent another glorious week cruising the islands. Michael thoroughly enjoyed this commission and met some lovely people. But he also found loads of problems, which actually put the safety of the passengers at risk. It was so frustrating for him to learn later that the charity didn't have the funds available to implement the recommended adjustments filed in his report. So why did they employ him for two weeks? It just didn't make sense.

Before he'd embarked on that trip, Michael had decided to once again move to bigger offices. His wife, Sue, had given up her accountants role and had taken over from Michael's mother to become the general manager of the business. With husband and wife working together, one can imagine that they didn't always see eye to eye when it came to how to run the business. Despite their disagreements, they made it work, and with Sue running things, the business actually prospered. Michael was then freed up to do what he was good at, leaving Sue to do all the things she was good at, including the admin, which Michael had been doing when his mum stopped working for him.

Moving from a 900-square-foot office to a unit of 2,800 square feet, they then needed to expand the workforce and the storage space. Looking after 400 or so ships from lots of clients, plus the hugely successful sales of up-to-date but pre-owned navigation charts, which were as good as brand new but 40 per cent cheaper than new ones, space was definitely at the top of Michael's requirements list.

Michael was able to reduce the number of charts carried by many of his clients' vessels, bringing the surplus back for storage and reuse on other vessels within their fleet. Effectively, he could reduce a chart outfit from 2,000 charts to about 1,000 charts, thereby landing the other 1,000. When applied to 10 or 20 ships in a fleet, this meant huge savings. Not just in the wasted time spent updating charts on board that were never going to be used, but it saved the company the cost of replacing outdated charts with new ones when they were published. It also meant that the company had a 20,000 chart stockpile at Marine Chart Services offices, which were then called upon for them to update and send extra charts to other ships whenever a new voyage required it. Only charging for the cost of the updates, it generally meant a company was getting the charts for £3/£4 instead of buying them at over £20 new, as had previously been the case. The United Kingdom Hydrographic Office didn't like Michael's venture one little bit because every chart MCS recycled meant a loss of £20-plus revenue for them. Michael never got a Christmas card from them. He wonders why?

Moving to bigger premises in 2001 was a good move in many ways, but not so good in another way, as the landlord was, as Michael eloquently explained, "A twat who made silly rules and micromanaged everything." Needless to say, they soon fell out and Michael had to get solicitors in to sort out the problems the landlord created. Staying there for the requisite five years minimum that the lease demanded was more than enough for Michael.

In May 2006 he moved MCS 250 yards along the road to their new premises, the aptly named by Michael, Maritime House. It was 4,300 square feet and gave them even more room to expand. Michael had developed a remote-access computer program that allowed ships at sea, anywhere in the world, to log into the MCS server and download critical navigation updates. They weren't the only company doing this, but it meant that they were still at the forefront of providing critical safety compliant services.

That same year, Michael won a contract with a large tugboat company that wanted him to devise a system that would keep all their vessels up to date for the charts held on board, as well as to develop a system that allowed them quick access to a set of charts that could take them anywhere in Europe at short notice. Michael was good at project management, and this task was a test of his skills. In collaboration with the operational managers, he came up with a cost-effective plan that they readily accepted. With nearly 80 vessels, it took Michael's team three months to implement the new system, and once in place and fully operational it was soon accepted by the various crews, and the company too. It was a lot of work, but also a good income generator.

With work not only floating but soaring, Michael's attention turned back to more personal matters. Knowing he was intersex had always been at the back of his mind, and in 2006 he decided he wanted to be female full time.

He approached his doctor and explained his feelings. She was very sympathetic and quickly referred him to the Northampton Gender Clinic. At that time, it had 43 patients, including Michael, and was situated in Campbell House near to Northampton's town centre. Michael's first appointment soon came, and in a flashback to boarding his third ship, unsure of how he should present himself, he went shopping. Kitted out in ladies' trousers, blouse and stiletto boots, he hobbled from the public car park to the entrance, as he couldn't walk in high heels. The clothing wasn't a problem, but the boots!! He sat at the edge of the general waiting area, feeling very self-conscious and thinking to himself, What a twat for wearing this lot! When he finally got to see the gender specialist, he was immediately put at ease.

The Northampton Gender Clinic was a satellite of the Nottingham Gender Identity Clinic, and it was there that Michael was being referred on to. He travelled to his first appointment in Nottingham by train and recalls getting a taxi to the clinic, but everything else is a blur.

Towards the end of 2007 Michael was struck down with the C. diff bug, and because he had started passing blood was taken by ambulance to Kettering General Hospital. He spent about five days in an isolation room before being transferred to a room off the general ward where he was to properly recover. The isolation and the seemingly poor attention of being in a single room really got to Michael, and feeling vexed he decided enough was enough. He pulled out the canula inserted into his wrist, took 25 mg of Warfarin (3 mg was a normal dose) and started to walk through the ward to go home. When the duty nurse noticed a bloody trail and saw the blood gushing out of his arm, she immediately stopped him, called for help and ushered him back into his room. With his bleeding wrist bandaged, Michael was told in no uncertain terms how foolish he had been to take the Warfarin, which he'd effectively overdosed on. He could have died. Weary with his world, Michael knew that could happen, but at the time didn't much care.

Part Four

Michelle

Chapter 21

To Section or Not to Section? That is the Question

ALL MEDICATIONS AND SHARP objects were removed from Michael's room and the consultant in charge of the ward was bleeped. Michael was soon getting another ear-bashing for what he had done. The consultant also told him that as he had deliberately overdosed, he had to be questioned by the mental health team. It would be about four hours before they could attend. Though the staff tried to make him feel stupid for what he'd done, Michael wasn't having any of it. He knew what he'd done and what the consequences could be.

To counteract the 25 mg of Warfarin he had taken, Michael was given a vitamin K tablet to swallow. Vitamin K reverses the effect of Warfarin, meaning that he wouldn't die after all. Looking back, Michael realises that he didn't really care. His overdose was in some ways a protest at being in isolation. He doesn't think he'd intended to kill himself.

Four hours soon passed and a team of people, including a social worker, a medical doctor, a psychiatric nurse and two people from the mental health crisis team, gathered in his room. Michael didn't know it at the time, but they were looking to see if he had lost capacity and needed to be sectioned under the Mental Health Act. They asked him lots of questions, mostly around why he had overdosed and what his intentions were. Michael answered truthfully and it was decided that he still had capacity and didn't need to be sectioned. The consultant of the ward was very disappointed when he was given the news, but he had no intentions of letting Michael stay on the ward, so he was discharged that evening.

Returning home was a big relief for Michael—so fed up was he of hospitals and isolation. However, his mental health became an issue, and within a month of being discharged he became very depressed. So much so that he couldn't stop crying. Sue was out of her depth and didn't know how to help her husband. Eventually, Michael contacted his GP, who referred him to the crisis team. After a lengthy chat with them, it was decided that Michael should spend some time in the local mental ill-health hospital—The Welland Centre (part of St. Mary's Hospital in Kettering).

Sue took him to The Welland, where he was admitted onto Kingfisher Ward. All his belongings were itemised and searched to make sure he hadn't brought any unwanted medicines or knives with him. Once he had been formally admitted, Michael was shown to his room—a single-bedded en suite.

Shown around the communal areas by a care assistant, M, who later became a good friend, Michael was informed of the relevant housekeeping. Medications would be dispensed around 8 am and 9.30 pm every day. Communal breakfast was available from 7.30 until about 9 am, and he should aim to be there for around 8 am. The dining area was part of the main room, which also had a large TV, several sofas and lots of chairs around the sides. Doors led to a small patio and garden. The patio was for use only at agreed times, and the doors were kept locked in between. The main doors into the ward were kept locked as well.

All staff carried emergency alarm buttons so that if any 'resident' kicked off, they could quickly summon help. Within the building were two other wards upstairs—one male and one female—and an intensive-care section. Each ward had an office where staff could monitor what was going on in their section, and they had use of several computers. The ward itself always had three or four members of staff interacting with the 'residents', as well as one or two staff in the office.

Although he was relatively sane, Michael knew he was very depressed and needed help. His depression got the better of him sometimes, and he can remember bending the prongs on a metal fork to insert it into an electrical socket in his room with the intention of electrocuting himself. Fortunately, once he'd inserted it into the socket and switched the switch to on, all the fuses blew. Michael didn't hurt himself, but it did mean he was put into the padded room for a couple of hours to 'reflect' on his actions.

On another occasion he took the CO_2 fire extinguisher from the wall near to his room and was in the process of trying to gas himself, having put the nozzle into his mouth, when a nurse who had seen him take the extinguisher burst into his room and extracted it from him. After a further period of time to 'reflect',

Michael was allowed back into his room. He had to pay £10 for the extinguisher to be recharged.

Michael's days were filled with occupational activities, like mindfulness, relaxation classes, craft groups, painting or reading. He was seen by a psychiatrist every couple of days, and she—Dr L—arranged for him to undergo some tests to see if he had Asperger's Syndrome. He was borderline. Michael was also seen and assessed by Team 63, who were tasked with finding out what was wrong with him. In the end they concurred that he had suffered mentally because of his heart attack. They thought that Michael was unable to accept that he had had a heart attack and that fact was causing his depression—a condition they called adjustment disorder.

Chapter 22

'M' for Michelle

MICHAEL'S STAY AT THE Welland lasted two weeks, after which he was discharged home. Though he was fit to go home, he wasn't really in a very good place and was still very depressed. Sue, bless her, did her best to cheer him up, but it didn't work. Going back to the office helped, as it kept Michael busy, so he didn't really have time to dwell and be unhappy.

Outside of work was a different matter. Depression ruled him. Often bursting into tears for no reason, Michael turned to self-harm to try to take the pain in his head away. Replacing it with the real pain of cutting his forearms worked, but it was only temporary relief.

It wasn't long before he was re-admitted to The Welland. His stays were relatively short, just three or four days each time, but during 2008 those stays were many. On one occasion it was suggested that Michael spent three days in a halfway house in Kettering. So after being discharged home, he was then accepted at Meadhurst on a Friday evening. The house had seven residents including Michael and was staffed by mental health workers who watched over the patients but didn't generally interact with them. Michael and his housemates had their own food, so were responsible for cooking and feeding themselves. With these everyday tasks designed to help the patients reintegrate into a more normal routine, help was immediately available should they have needed it. Of the seven patients, Michael was the only one with his own transport.

Though things were better in this controlled environment, depression still got the better of Michael. Even after a Sunday lunch which Michael generously paid for for everyone, he dropped into a very low mood and began cutting his arms again. He wasn't proud of what he did, but it did help him briefly, so he didn't tell the staff. But as the afternoon wore on, he decided he'd had enough and overdosed on the prescribed medications he had with him. Realising that he hadn't been seen in the communal areas for some time, a member of staff stopped by Michael's room and caught him in the act of overdosing. Michael's tablets were quickly confiscated, his pocket-knife removed and help was summoned.

Whilst his bleeding arms were bandaged, the crisis team, including a doctor and social worker, were called. After a brief chat with Michael, he was sectioned under the Mental Health Act.

Told to pack his gear away and leave his car keys with the staff, he learned he was being admitted to Berrywood Mental Hospital in Northampton but wasn't allowed to make his own way there. Instead, an ambulance was called, and Michael travelled the 18 or so miles in the ambulance, with a mental health nurse following in their car. Driving through Northampton Town Centre, Michael got severe chest pains and was hooked up to a monitor, which showed some irregularities. The paramedics radioed ambulance control to ask if they should take him to A&E or continue on to Berrywood. After a short while the controller said to carry on to the mental hospital, but to use blues and twos to get there. Quite what the nurse who was following thought, Michael really didn't know. The lights and sirens got him through Northampton and into the general area where the hospital was, but the crew couldn't find the hospital and had to stop several times to ask for directions. Berrywood was a relatively new hospital at the time on the outskirts of a new housing estate, and the driver didn't know which road to take. When they eventually arrived, the nurse that had been following had got there before them.

Berrywood was similar in make up to The Welland Centre. The admissions ward—Harbour Ward—had around 12 single bedrooms all with en suites. The bedrooms and bathrooms were bigger and more modern. The shower was actually a wet room. Central to the ward was a glass-fronted office, like in Kettering but the dining room and TV lounge were separate rooms. There was also a dispensary and a quiet room.

Michael's section was for two weeks, with a review scheduled at the end of the fortnight. During that time his movements were restricted. He wasn't allowed out without a nurse escort. As he was in the process of transitioning from Michael to Michelle, he asked to be called Michelle, but the staff refused. Consequently, Michelle asked to see an advocate. The lady who saw her was not amused at the staff's refusal to call her by her preferred name and made it very clear to them that it was Michelle's basic right to be called by the name of her choice. And so Michael became known as Michelle.

The two weeks' section soon passed, and the ward psychiatrist spoke to Michelle at length and agreed that she was to be allowed her relative freedom. The section was lifted. That didn't mean she could be discharged. Quite the opposite. Her stay at Berrywood lasted about four weeks, after which a bed became available at The Welland and Michelle was transferred back to Kettering.

Just before her transfer back, Michelle had tried to self-harm in her wet room, so the staff locked the door, meaning she had to ask to use the toilet. To her knowledge it was an unlawful act, as everyone has the right to use a toilet whenever necessary. Michelle made her grievance known by emptying her catheter bag on the carpet in a communal corridor. The staff were far from pleased with her, but it did the trick and the bathroom was unlocked.

Her transfer back to Kettering was uneventful, but the psychiatrist whose care she was under wouldn't discharge her home. In the end Michelle spent five months in the hospital, right through Christmas and New Year 2009.

During her transition, Michelle had regular appointments at the Nottingham Gender Identity Clinic. As she was not allowed out without an escort, it meant that she had to catch a train to Nottingham with a nurse. On one occasion, because they were too early for Michelle's appointment, they went to a nearby café. A gentleman who was about to leave stood up from his table and said, "Would you two ladies like my table?" Michelle was well chuffed.

As well as going to Nottingham, Michelle was also under the care of the Churchill Hospital, part of the John Radcliffe in Oxford, and the NHS kindly paid for her taxi there and back, again with a nurse escort. This was for her Klinefelter Syndrome, for which she had appointments roughly once each year.

Michelle spent most of her days in The Welland doing nothing, as there was only so much TV that she wanted to watch and the books she'd taken with her had all been read. As she didn't like playing scrabble all the time, she spent much of the time doing very little. She was allowed the use of her mobile phone, but the building was built in such a way that signals couldn't penetrate through to the communal lounge, so she had to go out onto the patio every two hours with the smokers, when they were allowed out, so that she could keep in touch with her office and support Sue in keeping the business running. In Michelle's absence, Sue did a magnificent job, keeping everything going and only referring to Michelle when it became absolutely necessary. Sue had picked up a little bit of shipping knowledge from talking to Mich before she finally left accountancy and worked for him. Michelle certainly couldn't have managed without her—for her business and for her welfare. Sue would visit Michelle almost every evening, which Michelle acknowledges must have been a terrible strain for her.

Towards the end of her six months' incarceration, Michelle was allowed out with Sue for short periods of time. So on some evenings they went for a nice steak meal at a restaurant in Kettering Town Centre. Getting out of the hospital was very good for Michelle, and for Sue, because it meant things were getting back to normal.

Having learnt some tips in hospital on how to overcome her sadness and be more positive, Michelle was finally, after one month in Berrywood and five months in The Welland, discharged home. Despite what she had learnt, she chose to seek private help and visited a hypnotherapist regularly, who taught her the art of self-hypnosis. This was beneficial for Michelle, as it meant she could hypnotise herself whenever her mood dipped, and it kept her from self-harming.

Chapter 23

Separation

MICHELLE'S RETURN TO 'normal' life was carefully monitored by the psychiatrist assigned to her at the Redcliffe Mental Health Clinic in Hatton Park Road, Wellingborough. Not long after being discharged from The Welland, Michelle was put on an antidepressant she hadn't heard of before: quetiapine (actually an antipsychotic drug which can occasionally be used as an antidepressant). Soon after she started taking these, Michelle's waistline began to increase. She doesn't remember that she was eating more, just that her waistline got bigger. At her three-month review, the psychiatrist told Michelle to stop taking this tablet, and when she asked why, she was told it was because her waist had become so large! "So what was the point in giving them to me in the first place?" Michelle scolded. Her waist had gone from a 34-inch to a 56-inch size in just three months! No wonder she was distraught at the news.

By stopping the tablets, Michelle reasonably assumed her waistline would decrease. It didn't. She read up on the tablets and found that virtually everyone who had taken them had reported excessive weight gain which was irreversible. If she had known that at the start of the course, Michelle would have refused to take them. A few years later she tried to lose weight by going to a gym three or four times a week. She lost weight, but not off her stomach. When the gym found out that she was on Warfarin, she was asked to leave, as it was against their policy to allow someone on blood-thinning medication to use their equipment. It seemed that now Michelle was stuck with a skinny body and a fat stomach. Ugh! Gross! She hated it. She tried to take legal action against the psychiatrist for prescribing the tablets, as she was not psychotic, but then found out that they could be used as an antidepressant, and the firm of solicitors she had approached refused to take the case on.

Over the next couple of years Michelle spent many days in The Welland Centre, mostly for five or six days at a time, although there was another six-month spell again over the Christmas and New Year period. By 2011 Michelle's mental stability improved and she was free of needing to be incarcerated. Not long into 2011 the cruise ship, *Costa Concordia*, hit some rocks off the coast of Italy and sank, causing some passengers to lose their lives. This was a 'hot' news topic, and as Michelle had a reputation for being a marine expert, she was contacted by BBC Radio Northampton for a live interview around why the ship had sunk. Though she managed to sound cool and calm in the radio interview, she was actually still quite fragile. Her daily workload was very basic, as she found it hard to concentrate, so Sue kept her doing menial tasks to help her refocus. Michelle didn't like this one little bit; however, knowing it was in her best interests, she went along with it.

By 2012 Michelle was back to 'normal'. Her life, and her gross belly, continued a normal working pattern. In November 2015, however, her marriage broke down badly. In an attempt to save their marriage, Michelle and Sue agreed to visit Relate, the marriage guidance service. Sadly, all this achieved was a flat refusal by Sue, who shared that she had been unhappy with their relationship for some 12 months, to even consider them staying together. Michelle found this hard to accept, as during the previous 12 months they had done some great things together and had both enjoyed themselves. Michelle was devastated. They had been married for over 31 years.

Sue insisted that Michelle found alternative accommodation, as she didn't want her in the house. Not knowing what to do or where to go, Michelle packed a suitcase and checked into a nearby three-star hotel. Her mother and stepfather were in their holiday home in Spain at the time though, and when Michelle finally revealed to her mum what had happened, she immediately told her to move into her house whilst they were in Spain. Knowing that her mother and stepfather had planned to stay in Spain until May, Michelle had the house to herself for as long as she wanted within that time frame. After living at her mum's for about six weeks though, Michelle came to her senses and realised that the marital home in Earls Barton was as much hers as it was Sue's. So she let her know she was moving back in, whether Sue liked it or not.

To say it was difficult would be an understatement. The breakdown of her marriage hit Michelle like a sledgehammer, and since she struggled to hold it together when they were apart, being under the same roof was intolerable.

Before Michelle moved back in, they'd previously booked a Twixmas break at a hotel in North Wales, so they decided to still go for the break, staying in two single rooms instead of the double they had reserved. Michelle had not long taken delivery of a new Mercedes Benz E-Class, which made the trip to Wales very smooth, though they barely spoke a word to each other except for checking directions. On arrival they each went to their own rooms and then met up in the bar to enjoy a festive drink, albeit at a high price. Having also prebooked a one-hour spa session, they both took it and then got ready for their evening meal. They must have been the only table at dinner that wasn't speaking. Outside after dinner, Sue insisted that she couldn't continue with the break and would go by taxi to the nearest station and a get train home.

Already being in a bad way mentally, the thought of being isolated in that hotel for another three days didn't sit well with Michelle. So, after a lot of arguing, they agreed they would both check out the next morning and Michelle would drive them back home. After dropping Sue off, Michelle made her way back to her mum's house in Wellingborough. She was suicidally depressed, but this time didn't act on her thoughts or feelings.

For some reason Sue invited Michelle for dinner on New Year's Day 2016. Whilst there, she all of a sudden got a blinding headache. It was so severe that she couldn't do anything, and none of her migraine painkillers worked. Still in terrible pain after about an hour or so, Michelle called 111 for help and was sent an ambulance. After checking her blood pressure, oxygen levels and doing a heart trace, the paramedics shifted up a gear. Fearing Michelle was having a bleed on the brain and needing urgent medical intervention, they sped her away in the ambulance with Sue following behind in her car.

At Northampton General Hospital, Michelle was given CT and MRI scans, both of which were normal. When the consultant asked about Michelle's lifestyle and heard what had happened, he concluded that she was suffering from a thunderclap headache brought on by stress.

Returning home with Sue, they continued a very difficult life under the same roof. Though Sue seemed to be coping well, Michelle wasn't. By March she had grown seriously suicidal and was again under the care of the mental health services. Consequently, around the middle of March 2016, she was re-admitted into The Welland Centre by the crisis team's psychiatrist for her own protection. After being in there for two weeks she was reassessed by the duty psychiatrist who then discharged Michelle that day. It was Good Friday. Michelle was beside herself, but her vehement protests at how suicidal she felt went unheard. A few hours later she was kicked out.

Michelle felt so desperately sad and depressed that she drove back to Earls Barton in tears. On the way she phoned the crisis team to seek help, but they said they couldn't overturn her discharge. In desperation she called BUPA, as she still had her membership from when she was in the Merchant Navy. Having explained to the lady what had happened and how desperate she was, Michelle was told not to worry, as BUPA had access to around 120 mental hospitals in the UK and she felt sure Michelle would soon be offered a bed. However, it was a bank holiday weekend, so nothing would happen until the Tuesday.

It took ages to get to Tuesday, but when it came, BUPA soon called Michelle with news of what they could offer her. Out of their 120 hospitals, only three would accept Michelle because of her high suicidal state. By this time it was 11 am, and the nearest hospital in North London would accept Michelle if she could get there by 1 pm. As she needed to go home and pack a case and stuff, then fill up her car with diesel before driving to and through North London, Michelle realised it just wasn't realistic. So now she had two hospitals to choose from: one in the centre of Manchester and the other in Brighton. Whichever one she chose, Michelle had to be there by 6.30 pm. She didn't like the thought of driving through Manchester, so agreed that she would be at The Priory Hospital in Brighton by no later than 6.30 pm.

Reckoning that, allowing for traffic, it would be a three- to four-hour drive, she calculated that she should easily be there by the deadline. So she left the office, went home, packed her stuff and set out for Brighton at around 1 pm. Despite having a big, comfortable and fast car, it took her until 6.15 pm to get there—just in time.

Before they would admit her, Michelle had to be assessed by the hospital's psychiatrist. He spoke with her for over an hour. Had he have known, he said, how bad she was before she had left home, he would have refused to accept Michelle, but since she was there, he had no choice but to do so. Being at such a high risk of self-harm or suicide, Michelle was given one of their two high-risk bedrooms directly overlooked by the nurses' station.

Chapter 24

All Things Brighton and BUPAful

MICHELLE'S ROOM WAS MUCH nicer than any of the NHS hospital rooms she'd previously been given, but then at £950 per night one would expect something better! With plush wall-to-wall carpet, a 26-inch TV, a large double bed with a sumptuous quilt, and a state-of-the-art en suite, it was equipped with emergency call buttons in each area. There was also a telephone so Michelle could easily contact room service to order meals 'to die for' from the permanent chef. Any patient occupying one of the 15 rooms, could order tea, coffee, soft drinks and snacks 24 hours a day. And the dining room was plush—not unlike a nice restaurant. In the mornings self-service cereals, toast and juice were available and a cooked breakfast was on offer if you wanted it. Lunch and dinner were three or four courses and very posh nosh. It reminded Michelle of happy times spent amongst the Indian crew on many of the Reardon Smith ships. Such a difference to the, wonderful though they are, NHS rooms where the beds had sheets and blankets, the floors were bare wood or covered in cheap carpets and you had to make your own bed.

Because Michelle was the highest risk patient in the hospital, she was put on fifteen-minute obs. It meant that a staff member had to be within arm's distance of her every quarter of an hour, day and night. Daytime wasn't a problem for Michelle, but as the doors in the Victorian house were heavy oak and Michelle's squeaked when opened or closed, night-time took a bit of getting used to. When the staff went into her room each time, they had to shine a torch onto Michelle to make sure she was breathing. It was hard for Michelle to do anything but, as she certainly wasn't getting much sleep!

Although she had driven to Brighton and her car was in one of the hospital car park's three spaces, Michelle was not allowed to use it. Initially, she was not allowed out of the building, but after her first three days, she was allowed into the garden with a close escort. At some time during the first few days someone caused the fire alarms to sound and the building was evacuated at 7.30 am. Michelle was having a shower at the time, and, as she didn't own a dressing gown, she had to quickly dry off and get dressed in order to get to the muster point. When she did get there, she was the last person to be accounted for and the fire engines were already in attendance. The fire turned out to be an electrical fault, and once the fire brigade had made sure everything was safe, everyone was allowed back in.

At the end of that first week, Michelle was given permission to walk into town, but with two nurses as escorts. The first thing to buy on her shopping list was a dressing gown, so she ventured into a ladieswear shop, accompanied by her two escorts. Though she knew she was a suicide risk, Michelle also knew that she wouldn't jump under a bus to kill herself—not then and not now. So having a double escort every time she wanted to go out was, she felt, a bit over the top.

As with all mental hospitals, when Michelle first arrived at the Brighton clinic, her belongings were catalogued and checked for blades of any sorts, scissors and anything else that could be used to self-harm, or worse. However, when you are desperate to self-harm, you get very clever at beating the system. Why did Michelle self-harm you may ask? By cutting her arms, it created a real pain that she could focus on, thereby relieving the pain in her head, or her mind, that cannot be touched. Hurting herself was a release of the terrible mental pain she experienced.

During the first week, she attended relaxation classes and just relaxed—if one can relax with terrible mental torment—into her surroundings. On the Monday of the second week, Michelle was asked to attend CBT (cognitive behaviour therapy) classes, where she would be involved in talking therapies. She recalls that there were only five or six patients in that group. Many of the others were recovering drug addicts for whom CBT wasn't appropriate. The talking therapy was meant to give patients time to reflect on their problems and try to understand their behaviours. However, this had the opposite effect on Michelle, and she became very distressed and suicidal in the group. Her distress affected the other group members, and the staff were unable to cope. CBT classes were held every Monday and Thursday, followed by relaxation classes, but at the end of the second class Michelle was told by the ward matron that she must not attend any more sessions. No reason was given. She was just told to stay away. Of course, that didn't sit well with Michelle, as she was at the hospital for treatment, and CBT was the treatment on offer. Consequently, on the Monday of the third week, session three, she joined the class again. When the therapist came in and saw her, she walked out again. Returning with two nurses, Michelle was expelled from the group.

Hoping for an explanation, Michelle went back to her room and relaxed in one of the armchairs. Monday passed, as did Tuesday and Wednesday, with no explanation. So, on the Thursday, Michelle told the services manager that she was leaving the hospital. When asked why, she explained about not being allowed to attend the classes. The services manager explained that access to the classes had been refused because her distress upset the other patients to the point that each needed one-to-one counselling. They simply didn't have the staff to cope, so Michelle had been prevented from attending. When she asked why she wasn't told this before, the manager just dismissed it. She went on to say that the psychotherapist would see Michelle on a one-to-one basis instead of her joining the group, which would give her the opportunity to talk about her feelings and help her manage the destructive thoughts she was having. She also said that had Michelle tried to leave, she would have been sectioned, as she was too dangerous to be allowed out on her own.

Though she was regularly in tears within 10 minutes of starting therapy and the psychotherapist brought out some of Michelle's worst feelings, she got on well with her during the hour-long, twice-weekly sessions. But after each session Michelle would feel really low and the mental pain was again unbearable. Desperate people do desperate things. Michelle had secreted away lancets she used for testing her blood-clotting levels in her bags and used these to carve into her arms or wrists to create the physical pain she needed. She was always given first aid pretty soon after cutting herself, as she was still on fifteen-minute observations, but at the end of her stay the psychotherapist told Michelle that she needed to find somewhere that did DBT (dialective behaviour therapy), as this was the treatment for her condition. She had diagnosed Michelle as having a personality disorder.

With some physical health needs that needed looking after whilst she was in Brighton, Michelle was driven to 'proper' hospitals to attend to these—her two escorts closely by her side on each occasion. In an attempt to give her some outside interest, the staff found out that the local gay community—let's face it, Brighton *is* the gay capital—held a trans drop-in and coffee shop in a building in town. With her two 'sidekicks', Michelle pitched up at the building and went in. Well! What a seedy place it was. A trans place it was indeed, but not one for transsexuals like Michelle, but for transvestites (people who dress as the opposite gender on a part-time basis). Michelle remembers there was an oldish guy dressed in a white blouse, with a massive fake chest and tight-fitting leather skirt with heels. He made her cringe. He clearly got kicks out of the way he was dressed, which is why Michelle has little time for transvestites. For her, transvestites, drag queens and others like them belittle everything that a true transgender person is trying to be. They do it for kicks, whereas Michelle, and people who are transitioning, do it because it is who they are. "A true trans person gets no sexual kick out of dressing the way I do—be it trans male or trans female," explains Michelle. Allowed to stay for two hours, Michelle got the nurses to call for transport within the first hour, as the group was not what she wanted, nor where she wanted to be. She willingly and warmly gives the hospital credit for trying though.

By the fourth week, Michelle was becoming concerned for her car. It hadn't been moved at all in that time and she didn't want to end up with a flat battery. Having relayed her concerns to her allocated nurse, and after some deliberations by the staff, she was advised that one of their colleagues would take her car out for a run. This was definitely not on. Not least because her car was worth around £40,000 and if they damaged it their insurance would only give third-party cover, leaving Michelle to pay for any damage to her vehicle, but also because cars were her pride and joy. She protested that this was not going to happen, and in the end was allowed to go out in it for an hour with one of the stronger male nurses in the passenger seat next to her. Regardless of the heavy, this was like a breath of fresh air to Michelle; she was allowed out in her car. Whoopee! But the hour soon passed and she was back in her comfy hospital room on fifteen-minute obs again.

Michelle made regular phone calls to her mother and stepdad using the free hospital landline. During one of these calls her stepdad told her they were going to drive down to Brighton in their motorhome and visit her. He said they would come down that weekend. This was so good to hear, as Michelle had had no visitors in the weeks she had been there. However, the weekend came and went, and no visitors arrived. When she phoned her mum again, L—her stepdad—answered and said they hadn't come down to see her because she had said something wrong in her last call to them that they weren't happy with. Michelle, to this day, has no idea what she was meant to have said, and her stepdad didn't elaborate, other than to say it was her 'punishment' for what she'd uttered. L came into Michelle's life in the year 2000, and she didn't much care for him then. She cared even less for him as she tried to imagine what on earth could have upset him and her mother so much. It is a sad truth that in all her previous admissions, her mum and stepdad rarely visited her. In each of the six-month stays, they only visited two or three times, even though they were only seven miles away.

Michelle's stay at The Priory was limited to the amount of funding put up by BUPA, and that funding came to an end after seven and a half weeks, meaning Michelle had used up her £50,000 allowance. Before she was allowed to leave she had to be assessed by the psychiatrist again. This took quite some time. In the end he pronounced that she wasn't fit to drive home, as she was still very suicidal. "But since you drove down in that state," he went on, "you should be able to drive back." At which point he signed Michelle's discharge papers and she was allowed to leave.

"My thanks," Michelle said afterwards, "go to BUPA for allowing me to stay in such plush surroundings for so long."

Chapter 25

Rebellion

ALTHOUGH THE PSYCHIATRIST at The Priory thought Michelle was at risk of causing an accident, her return journey was uneventful; after all, none of her suicide attempts had ever involved anyone else, and causing an accident was not on her agenda.

As she didn't want to go home to an empty house, she had organised, through a local agency, for a carer to be there to greet her. Michelle rang the agency when she left Brighton and called again when she was an hour away to ensure everything was set. However, when she finally arrived home in Earls Barton there was no one there. Already distraught because of her internal pain and suffering from her divorce, finding her house empty just made things 10 times worse. She called the agency and was told the carer would be with her in 30 minutes. Michelle was not a happy bunny! She had also requested a hot evening meal on her arrival home and for the following three days, but the agency couldn't even get *that* right. On the second evening, the food arrived cold, and on the third it didn't arrive at all.

Though she doesn't remember everything following her return home, Michelle does remember going to work a week or so later, only to find that one of her staff, who was persistently late despite numerous warnings, had not arrived. She turned up after 30 minutes with no acceptable excuse. Michelle berated her for her continual lateness, and she ended up shouting at Michelle as though it was her fault! Being so terribly fragile, this plunged Michelle into suicide mode. She left the office in tears, took an overdose of tablets then went to her car to get more. Fearing for her welfare, one of the other staff members managed to wrestle some of the medication from Michelle, but still holding onto some, she drove off. She was so upset and angry, that her overwhelming feeling was that she just didn't want to be on this planet any longer.

She drove to a quiet country lane and parked in a farm entrance and just sat there crying. Then her phone rang with an unknown caller ID. She recalls that she foolishly answered it, to find it was the police asking where she was. Concerned, they told Michelle to return to her office to get help. As this wasn't what she wanted, she ended the call. Thinking that the police would have traced the call to find out where she was, Michelle drove off towards the Irchester Country Park and parked between some lorries, so she couldn't be easily seen, in a nearby lay-by. Then she took more tablets. The police rang again, but Michelle just told them it was too late, as she'd already overdosed, and ended the call.

Sitting in her car waiting for the overdose to kick in, all of a sudden two police cars with lights and sirens blaring turned up. As her phone call had been for less than a minute, Michelle couldn't understand how they had found her so quickly. An officer nearest to the car reached in through the driver's window, which was open three or four inches, and grabbed the ignition key. They then opened the door and hauled Michelle out. Four officers were in attendance, two of them were reasonable—good cops—but the other two were not. They were the bad cops whose tactics could have been straight out of a movie when they snarled, "Cuff her!" The good cops obviously realised how delicate the situation was and instead just put Michelle into the back of one of the cars. She was then driven at very high speed, with blues and twos, towards Northampton General Hospital. Speeding along at 120 mph, Michelle remembers at one point a van blocking their route, yet the police driver didn't slow down. She shouted, "You're going to kill me!" to which they retorted, "That was what you wanted!" At the last second, the van pulled over and the police car, with Michelle crouching in the corner, zoomed onwards down the A45. Though crazy thoughts were whizzing through her head, she recalls thinking sadly that her own car was being impounded.

After checking in at the hospital, Michelle asked the officers how they had found her. It turned out that her office had supplied her car details, including registration, and—via Mercedes support—they had found the location pinpointed by the satellite system and locator embedded into all new Mercedes cars. Michelle was so mad that she hadn't thought of this herself.

Michelle remained in hospital for three or four days, but luckily wasn't sectioned. Not long afterwards, the Northamptonshire NHS Foundation Trust appointed a mental health nurse/care coordinator to her, with whom she had weekly appointments. Michelle didn't really take to KT, as she thought she was quite bolshy and dictatorial. However, in August 2016, when Michelle was at a particularly low ebb, she suggested she spend five days in The Warren, a new 'crisis safe house' in Northampton, for some respite away from life's stresses and to give her space to try and feel better.

Michelle booked into the very large seven-bedroom—no en suites—bungalow and quickly figured out that breakfast and hot or cold drinks could be made in the communal kitchen. Though she can't be sure, she thinks the main meals were prepared by other patients and there were always two or three staff on duty 24/7. Michelle palled up with a female patient and they became friends. Explaining that she wanted to get out of her parents' house in Corby and find somewhere to live and rebuild her life, Michelle—foolishly in hindsight—let her move into a separate room in her house.

Things did not go well, and when her new friend started to rule her life, Michelle kicked her out. Hoping, she thinks, for a relationship to happen, Michelle had by then spent nearly £1,000 indulging her demands. That it didn't was clearly a good thing. KT was not happy with Michelle's housemate and repeatedly suggested that Michelle give her notice to move out. At the time, Michelle couldn't see how harmful the liaison was to her well-being, but common sense prevailed in the long run. But Michelle was still desperately sad and lonely when she left. All her life there had always been someone around her. As a child it was her family, in the Merchant Navy her shipmates, then in her marriage her wife. Now there was no one, and she couldn't deal with it. To this day—early 2021—she is still alone, but more in control.

She continued to see KT every week, and her dislike for her waned. When they were first introduced, Michelle was with a doctor's practice in Earls Barton. They had put her onto daily prescriptions to try to stop her from overdosing. Prescriptions had been monthly before that, and Michelle was not amused by having to collect a prescription every day. So much so that she rebelled against the system.

Because of the problems she had with blood clots, she had to take blood-thinning tablets (Warfarin) every day to keep her therapeutic. So to try to persuade her doctor to put her onto weekly prescriptions, or even fortnightly, she refused to collect each day's prescription. Unbeknownst to her doctor, she had a stash of Warfarin tablets hidden away so that she could in fact keep herself therapeutic. Unaware of this, the doctor got very angry with Michelle, declaring that she HAD to get her prescriptions or she could die. Hoping that he would increase the duration of her scripts, that was exactly what Michelle hoped he would think. It didn't work!

Michelle recalls how one day during her first week of rebellion, during a mental health assessment, she received a call from her doctor. He was beside himself with rage and was shouting down the phone to her so much that Michelle couldn't understand what he was saying. Instead, she passed the phone to the psychiatric doctor who was assessing her, who was able to calm the GP down enough to allow her to take note of what he was trying to say. In the end she was able to explain to Michelle that she was being kicked out of the surgery and would need to find another doctors' practice to take her on. This was not in Michelle's game plan! She had no choice but to accept daily prescriptions for the two or three weeks it took to find another practice that would accept her.

As there were only two doctors' practices in the village, she approached the other one and fortunately was accepted by them. However, that caused more problems, as they wanted to verify Michelle's identity. Though she had legally changed her name and bank account details in June 2016, her passport still said

Michael. As they wanted to see that her passport matched her gender identity, which it didn't, Michelle can remember several instances where she was misgendered because of this—something that can be quite emotionally damaging to a person who does not identify with the gender being prescribed to them. It wasn't until 2017 that Michelle was able to have her passport identity changed, as it requires supporting letters from the gender clinic, as well as declarations from Michelle to do this, which all took time.

Meanwhile, Michelle was experiencing problems with some of the medications she was given to control her mood. She was taking Valium (diazepam) most days, but it badly affected her coordination and driving. On one occasion she recollects driving down the A45 at around 75 mph in the right-hand lane and hitting the kerb of the central reservation and bouncing around the road. On another she turned a corner on her housing estate and ended up driving on the path on the opposite side of the road. The Valium was at the root of this dangerous driving, so when Michelle told KT about it, she inevitably reported it to the DVLA and Michelle's driving licence was revoked. Her dislike towards KT resurfaced, as she felt she had stepped beyond the boundary of looking after her. From then on Michelle either used the generosity of friends or paid for taxis.

Michelle's mental health assessment identified her as having EUPD (emotionally unstable personality disorder), the treatment for which was DBT. NHFT (Northamptonshire Healthcare NHS Foundation Trust) ran two courses of this treatment every week: one in Northampton and the other in Kettering. With the Northampton course being oversubscribed, the Kettering course was made available to her, and she entered into the programme around October 2016.

Well, what a load of crap that was!—or so Michelle thought. She remembers that in the third or fourth week, the patients were asked to sort a pile of coloured beads into piles of beads the same colour. Michelle couldn't believe that she—a trained captain—was actually messing with little beads. But she said nothing. The following week, they were asked to do some colouring onto sheets with outlines to make them look nice. That just about did it for Michelle, and she stood up, told them it was a load of crap and stormed out. She had to phone a friend and work colleague to pick her up, as she had no way of getting home and could hardly contain her rage at KT for proposing she joined the course.

Despite all of her negative feelings towards the care coordinator, KT continued working with her. She could see that her patient was progressing in her journey towards taming her destructive urges. Now, in 2021, Michelle is no longer under the care of the mental health teams, but KT is still a friend.

Chapter 26

999

Northamptonshire's mental health services run 'crisis cafés' in various locations around the county, and Michelle often went there for support. As they ran each day of the week, usually from around 7 to 10 pm, Michelle found these to be a safe place where she could talk to other people with mental health problems and bounce ideas. At the Kettering crisis café, held in the MIND charity building on Russell Street, she met and became casually acquainted with a girl who had similar mental health issues to her. However, she had spent a long time in a mental institution out of this county, where she had received 'inpatient' DBT treatment. She mentioned that there was a lot of crap in the course, but a lot of good things too. Seeing her every Wednesday or Thursday evening made Michelle realise that she had probably been a bit hasty in the judgement of the course she'd walked out of.

After discussing the pros and cons with her and one or two others, Michelle decided to ask KT if she could get her back into the treatment programme. KT thought this would be very difficult, because Michelle's departure had been viewed as final and they weren't keen to take her back. However, luck prevailed, and after several weeks it was agreed that Michelle could start over at the next opportunity in a couple of months.

Still without transport, as her licence had not been reissued by the DVLA, Michelle had no end of problems getting around. She hated being dependent on her friends and colleague, SA, to run her around, or having to pay for taxis when she had a perfectly good car sitting on her drive. To add to her troubles, in November and then again in December 2016, she suffered from two TIAs, or mini strokes, which left her with mobility and balance problems. She had begun attending another crisis café at the MIND building in Regent Square, Northampton, where, as well as Mind staff, there was also an NHS mental health nurse to turn to if needed. Michelle's care coordinator, KT, also regularly worked at the Northampton crisis café, which is how and where Michelle got to know her better.

KT suggested that Michelle should get a mobility scooter, but Michelle just felt that was giving in. Though she had a walking frame and extra support handles on the stairs, in the shower and by each toilet at home, she drew the line at anything more than the three-wheeled walker she reluctantly used to get to the crisis café with. Getting a mobility scooter somehow felt that she would never get back to normality, and that was her primary goal. KT also suggested that Michelle got herself a dog for companionship, but her old fear of dogs prevented her from doing that. Apart from anything else, she really couldn't see herself taking a dog for walks—not because of her mobility issues, but because she simply couldn't imagine picking up its pooh!

Sometime into 2017 Michelle decided that not having a driving licence wasn't going to stop her from getting about. She adopted a different mindset and new strategies that enabled her to get safely from A to B. Her emotional well-being began to improve until, as part of her DBT therapy, she was assigned another nurse, SM, who basically debriefed Michelle every week following her Tuesday DBT session. Whilst KT was good at sorting her out every couple of weeks, SM really got inside her head, regularly causing her to cry.

Although she was having DBT therapy, Michelle was still very suicidal and attended hospital by emergency ambulance on a regular basis. During a 12 month period covering 2016/17 she made over 40 suicide attempts, had over a hundred emergency attendances at Northampton General Hospital and many others to Kettering General Hospital. This placed her on the 'frequent attenders' list for the East Midlands Ambulance Service and they asked to meet with her, her doctor, the A&E consultant from Northampton General Hospital, KT and someone else to take notes.

This meeting took place at Michelle's GP practice in September 2017. She remembers it very clearly, as she was told that she regularly displayed her breast prosthesis to NGH hospital staff, which often caused distress to some of the younger nursing staff. Michelle found this very hard to accept, as she didn't consider this to be something she would do. It badly upset her. However, when she challenged the accusation, the A&E consultant, MP, produced a list of dates she had exposed her prosthesis. Michelle had a hard time processing this information. It just felt so out of character to her. She left the meeting feeling very distressed. Arriving home a few minutes later, still distraught, she ended up taking an overdose. Whatever had been said had made her feel so vulnerable that she imagined all sorts of scenarios including ending up in prison. The thought of her as a trans female in prison was unthinkable. She would be abused and raped, or worse. Not able to handle these terrifying thoughts, she did the only thing she felt was open to her and overdosed to end it all.

She came to her senses shortly afterwards, as she often did after taking an overdose, and called 999 for help. The ambulance whisked her away to NGH where she found that MP was the duty consultant. Asking why she had done it this time, Michelle told him it was because of what he had said to her in the earlier meeting. She doesn't recall much more about the incident and thinks she was in hospital for two or three days.

In some of her emergency admissions to NGH, Michelle was told she was going to be sectioned, so she regularly self-discharged to stop this happening. Once when she did this, a police car was sent to fetch her back at 4 am! Knowing that the law wouldn't allow her to be sectioned in her own house, when the police turned up, she refused to open the door. Unfortunately for Michelle, the officer was very stubborn and told her she had two minutes in which to open the door, after which he would kick it in. Michelle was driven back to hospital to face the consequences. On that occasion the hospital agreed not to section her if she would go voluntarily into Berrywood Mental Hospital in Northampton, which, of course, she did.

There were times when there were no beds available either at Berrywood or at The Welland Centre, and then Michelle was taken to the mental hospital in Milton Keynes. It had a much stricter regime and was nowhere near as 'nice' as the local hospitals, if one can say a mental hospital is ever nice. Other people in similar situations were taken to the nearest available hospital with a bed, and this was often hundreds of miles away. The system was such, though, that when a local bed became available, you were always shipped out back to Northamptonshire.

Chapter 27

A Cheerless Christmas

WITH HER VISITS FOR DBT and debriefs with her DBT nurse, SM, as well as working in the Marine Chart Services office, the weeks passed quickly for Michelle. The business was healthy, but Michelle had reached a point in her life where she had had enough of working long days and much of the weekends. The stress of having staff was also becoming a problem. Michelle reached a turning point when one staff member took issue with her being trans, as well as for her mental state. For their own health and safety as much as her own, Michelle had spoken to her staff members about what to do if she became suicidal, like calling an emergency ambulance or calling the police. Everyone accepted the potential risks of having to cope with their boss having a suicidal incident, except for one colleague: JL. Though he was gay and lived with his male partner, he took exception to Michelle's request for help in an emergency, even though as a diabetic he himself had advised his colleagues what to do should he become hypoglycemic. A stock of glucose tablets was on hand to give to him should it become an emergency. Somehow he didn't accept that if Michelle or his colleagues had to look after him in an emergency, then it was only reasonable to ask him and the other staff to look out for Michelle if she got into a crisis situation.

His lack of support dumbfounded Michelle and went, she thought, beyond reasonable. JL clearly didn't and filed a claim to the Industrial Tribunal on the grounds that his boss had been unreasonable in asking him to look out for her. Michelle didn't appoint a solicitor, as she felt sure the tribunal would kick the claim out—but they didn't! They actually agreed to take, what was to Michelle's mind, the frivolous and vexatious claim on. Michelle just couldn't believe it. She felt he was gunning for her because she was trans and had a mental health condition!

He left Michelle's employment, which made the working atmosphere better, as, though he was good at his job, his wimpishness created a different set of issues. The stress of the situation, coupled with the strain of running the office without a manager to help her, drove Michelle to downsize the business. She held a staff meeting and advised everyone that they would be made redundant in about three months' time. Though she was trying to be fair, she couldn't give a firm date at that point, as she was trying to sell the client lists and the ongoing contracts she had with them. One of her suppliers in Hull agreed to buy the contracts and client lists for a fixed sum up front, followed by a three-monthly commission percentage based upon the work generated by the clients. The commission was for five years on a reducing percentage each year. Once this was confirmed, Michelle was able to give notice of the termination date to her staff—for the end of June 2017.

Prior to the closure date, Michelle arranged for the buyer in Hull to collect the mountain of charts and publications her company was holding for their clients. It took them several visits in a van before they were finished. Once they had gone Michelle was tasked with selling off all the furniture and office equipment. She wasn't closing the business down, but was stopping all service work in favour of selling used charts and vintage charts via her own website and eBay shop. Having taken on a property measuring just 700 square feet, she had to reduce the quantity of used charts she owned, as she simply didn't have enough room to house them. With her staff gone to other employment, it was down to Michelle, a friend and the ex-employee, SA, to dismantle all the storage units and reassemble the ones she wanted to keep at the new premises in Northampton. Finally, the last thing to do, as the Wellingborough rental agreement cited, was to make good and redecorate the offices before leaving. Michelle was pleased when the landlord told her he intended to renovate the building, so she didn't have to worry about making good. Despite that, it still took until December 2017 before she had wiped out any trace of her or Marine Chart Services being there. Though the new business premises, which were in a shared industrial unit in Northampton, were only small, Michelle managed to get everything she needed set up in the smallish office and storage area and was pleased that all her racking and stock just about fitted in. Though he had another job as a night-shift packer in a warehouse, so could only give his friend a couple of hours work some mornings, she was also happy that her friend, SA, was able to continue helping her out with things whenever he could.

Whilst all this was going on, JL was still trying to get Michelle into court. On the first date the tribunal set, Michelle was unable to attend, as she had a medical procedure planned at Northampton General Hospital. On the second date, she was so distressed and suicidal that the tribunal agreed she was unfit to attend. And when the third date was set, JL called the case off, as he was in a bad way with his diabetes. Michelle knows she should have felt sorry for him, but that was the last thing on her mind; she was so thankful that it was all over. Even now, though, she still finds it hard to believe the tribunal accepted, what was in her mind, such a discriminatory case.

Michelle's mental health was still not brilliant, so she continued going to the crisis cafés, particularly the one in Northampton. On one of those visits, in November 2017, she met a girl called ZW, who, though about 20 years younger than Michelle, she particularly liked. They struck up a conversation but didn't exchange contact details. They got on well, but with no way of contacting her, other than to see if she returned to the crisis café, Michelle knew she had to be patient.

With Christmas coming up, that November KT suggested that Michelle go away over the Christmas and New Year period, as these were particularly difficult times for her. After some cajoling from her and others at the café, Michelle booked a triple break with Warner's Leisure Holidays at their hotel in Somerset, spending around £3000 for a stay over Christmas, Twixmas and the New Year. She was excited that this year would be different—not lonely like previous Christmas holidays—and as she was told when she booked that there would be other singles there and that many of the clients were in her age bracket, she had no reason to doubt it would be anything other.

When she arrived on 23 December, she found out otherwise. The average age of the 400 guests was in fact around 80, and many of them had mobility scooters which they used within the hotel complex. At dinner she found that there were only two other single people—not quite what she had been told. She considered herself lucky that the people on the table she was assigned to were not too old, and one was ex-Royal Navy, so they at least had a common talking point.

Despite this, Michelle felt very lonely, and it wasn't long before her mood plummeted and her thoughts turned to suicide. Before she could do anything, she suffered severe chest pains on Christmas Day afternoon. An ambulance was called and she was taken to the hospital in Taunton. With some relief, she was told that she hadn't had a heart attack, but more than likely an angina attack. So after an eye-watering £30 taxi ride, she was back at the hotel the next day. That evening she developed problems with her blood when a small cut wouldn't stop bleeding. As she was still bleeding the next day, she was once again taken to Taunton hospital for treatment. What they did, Michelle can't remember, but she clearly recalls that she had to pay for another £30 taxi ride back to the hotel later that day.

Her loneliness in the hotel, and the distress of going to hospital twice, was too much for Michelle to handle. Vulnerable and feeling lost, her thoughts again turned to suicide. It was around 28 or 29 December now and she'd had enough. Being lonely at home was bad enough, but being lonely in a hotel miles from home that had cost an arm and a leg was even worse. Michelle knows that she overdosed and is aware that the hotel called 999, but she doesn't remember much else. Returning to the hotel and escaping another hefty taxi fare, as the cost was covered by the hospital, she realised she'd had more than enough and decided to check out. The hotel management weren't happy about her leaving, so she explained how misled she'd been when she booked the break and how lonely and distressed she had become whilst there. Driving home on 30 December in a poor mental state was not ideal, but infinitely better than being in the hotel.

New Year's Day came and went, and on 2 January Michelle went back to work. But her troubles were not over. Though her new office was comparatively warm, she began shivering. She pulled her coat around her, but still couldn't get warm. She also began drifting in and out of consciousness. Alarmed, and with difficulty, she called for an ambulance. It took them a while to find her, as the area her unit was in was hard to locate from the road. When they finally arrived, the paramedics soon found that Michelle was suffering from hypothermia. She was wrapped in blankets and taken to Northampton General Hospital, where for the third time in as many weeks, she was kept in overnight.

The next day, and another taxi, she returned to the unit, where she retrieved her car and drove home. As she was still in a mental low, she returned to the crisis café, where she was told that ZW, the girl she had chatted to in November, had been asking after her. With still no way of contacting her, she continued to wait patiently and hope that she would soon come into the café. Fortunately, two or three more visits later she did.

Chapter 28

SCAM!

ON THE NEXT OCCASION that Michelle saw her, they chatted happily in the café. As things seemed to be going well, Michelle offered to drive ZW home. Protesting that it was only a short walk and would mean going out of Michelle's way, she refused, but Michelle being Michelle—kind and generous—wouldn't accept her refusal. So, she drove her the half mile back to her flat in Kingsthorpe, where they bade each other good night. On their next two meetings at the same café, the same thing happened, but on the third occasion, ZW invited Michelle over for a coffee the following Friday evening. ZW warned Michelle that her flat was a bit of a mess, but not being one to judge how other people live their lives, Michelle reassured her that it wouldn't bother her.

Friday came and, feeling excited, Michelle turned up at ZW's third-floor flat located in a small block. ZW's estimate of her messy flat was not exaggerated, but she'd cleared enough room for Michelle to sit down. With coffee on the go, ZW suggested Michelle might like to watch the documentary, *Transgender Street*, that had recently aired on TV and which she had missed. Keen to see it, they settled down to watch the documentary. It was an insightful watch for Michelle, as it followed the transition of two or three people who used the London Transgender Clinic (LTC) rather than the NHS route Michelle was taking. After a couple of hours, having had a pleasant evening, Michelle stood up to take her leave. Standing in the doorway, they had an awkward moment, with neither one of them knowing whether to hug or kiss or not. They did neither, and Michelle left.

The programme they had watched stayed with Michelle, and because she had not previously heard of the LTC, she contacted them to see if she would be able to have some surgery done through them. Michelle was still very unhappy about her increased waistline, a disastrous side effect from when she was prescribed quetiapine by her psychiatrist in 2009. No matter what she did, nine years later she still couldn't reduce her waist size, and she saw LTC as a possibility for having a tummy tuck.

Phoning them in January 2018, she was surprised and lucky enough to get an appointment in February at their clinic in Wimpole Street, near to Harley Street. Not wanting to go on her own, Michelle asked ZW if she would go with her, and they drove to London in plenty of time for Michelle's midday appointment.

The consultant, CI, was a very pleasant man, and after discussing Michelle's medical history and noting all the risks, he said he could perform the required surgery. Michelle returned home hopeful that soon her nightmare tummy would be gone. Her joy was so high that when the quote for the procedure came through a few days later, she accepted the cost of £12,000, even though it was double what she might have had to pay elsewhere. CI was after all, the first surgeon to consider the risks involved and still move forward with Michelle's requirements. Further appointments and tests followed, including an MRI of Michelle's stomach, a heart trace and echo and a lung function test at a London clinic—all of which added a further £1,000 to Michelle's costs. Nevertheless, it was a cost she was willing to accept, as it meant getting the surgery she so badly wanted.

Meanwhile, Michelle's relationship with ZW continued. It wasn't the easiest romantic liaison, as ZW also suffered with some quite serious mental health issues. They grew closer though, and ZW regularly stayed over at Michelle's house for a couple of days at a time, often in a separate room, which Michelle was sort of okay with.

Disappointment clouded Michelle's growing happiness when her surgery with the LTC, which should have taken place at a top private hospital in London around the end of 2018, didn't go ahead. For reasons unknown to Michelle, the hospital stopped her consultant from operating there, so her surgery was put on hold until another suitable hospital, with the kind of facilities Michelle's surgery needed, such as an intensive-care unit in case something went wrong, could be found.

Time spent waiting for them to obtain operating licenses went slowly, and in the end Michelle paid another £250 to see a female plastic surgeon who operated from the hospital that had stopped CI from practising. She had a clinic in Harley Street, and after an hour of talking to Michelle there, she refused to operate because she felt her patient was too high a risk. Michelle had no choice but to await news from LTC.

Michelle and ZW often went to other crisis cafés around the county, as their visits gave them both a safe place to be, with help on hand. On one occasion, knowing they were open until

10.30 pm, they went to the Wellingborough café at around 8.30 in the evening. On arrival, they were met by a MIND worker they knew called J, who told them that due to some issues over their payments, the café was having to close at 9.00 pm. This was not good news, as ZW was in a bad state and she badly needed to talk to a nurse.

At 9.00 pm Michelle and ZW sat outside in Michelle's car and talked for around 20 minutes, during which time the MIND staff, J included, left to go home. ZW decided that she wanted to get drunk, and though Michelle doesn't like to see people three sheets to the wind, on this occasion, knowing it was one of ZW's coping mechanisms, she drove her to Tesco to buy some wine.

Arriving back at Michelle's house at around 10 pm, ZW quickly drank about a third of a bottle then kicked off. She said she wanted to kill herself, which was not what Michelle wanted or needed to hear, and definitely not what she wanted her to do. No matter how much Michelle tried to calm and console her, ZW was adamant that she wanted to go home kill herself. Michelle was distraught, but knowing that it was not within her power to stop another person from ending it all, she drove her home to Northampton, crying all the way there and back. ZW's actions had a very negative effect on Michelle, who couldn't handle the thought of her special friend killing herself, and triggered her own feelings of suicide. She overdosed on heparin injections and tranquilisers.

As had happened on previous occasions, Michelle came to her senses after taking the near-lethal cocktail and called 999. The ambulance soon arrived, but other than knowing how she let them in, what happened afterwards is a blur caused by the high dose of tranquilisers she had taken. She does remember being taken from A&E and put into resuscitation—she was told for 12 hours—where she vaguely remembers a doctor saying that she didn't think she could save Michelle. Even though she had called the ambulance herself, the news that she might actually die made Michelle feel good. However, they saved her and she was transferred to a ward sometime later.

Heparin thins the blood, and a normal dose of 150 units was enough to maintain a healthy blood flow. However, Michelle had injected seven syringes—1,050 units—and her body didn't like it. Where she had injected them, around her waistline, was black and blue in a massive bruise, and her left arm went a violent purple colour. Michelle knows there is an antidote for heparin, but isn't sure how quickly it works. Her guess is that the heparin she'd taken had caused bleeding all over her body.

Michelle was in hospital for three or four days. Still concerned about ZW, she asked if her friend had been brought in, but was told she hadn't. Michelle messaged her and learnt that she had gone straight to bed that fateful night. Michelle was glad that she was still safe but reacted angrily to the news, as it felt like her antics had inadvertently caused her own near-death experience. ZW, on the other hand, didn't visit Michelle because she was angry with her for overdosing. They patched things up, and their friendship—not a relationship—continued. There were many other times that ZW kicked off, but Michelle had learnt not to rise to these events and instead just tried to calm her down. Throughout all of these times, Michelle was still waiting to hear from LTC that another hospital would accept her for surgery, but that news never came. She heard that LTC were trying to work with one other hospital, but after several months nothing came of it.

Christmas 2018 and New Year 2019 quickly passed and Michelle's friendship with ZW grew more precarious. Needing to find a more stable relationship instead of what had become just a casual friendship, Michelle enrolled with an online dating agency. In January 2019 she met Suzanna Shanks.[11]

Unbeknownst to Michelle, Suzanna was part of a very slick organised crime gang. Clearly experienced at seeking those most vulnerable, she wooed Michelle into believing they had something good going on . . . then slowly and gradually milked her out of her money. After handing over the first £1,000, Michelle wondered if she had been scammed and contacted the police. She was told that she was a victim of a romance scam and that she should have nothing more to do with Suzanna. Not seeing herself as that susceptible, Michelle wasn't convinced. Instead she checked out Suzanna's name against the various details she had given her. The money she had already given her was for a flight with KLM to New York, and when Michelle contacted the KLM desk, they confirmed that someone by that name did indeed fly with them. This made Michelle doubt what the police had said and believe Suzanna's story.

Michelle is a clever person who has many qualifications and areas of expertise. She has held positions of responsibility that include keeping people safe and healthy. Yet, as she says, like a fool, she kept handing money over in the knowledge that Suzanna was going to repay it. Whenever she had doubts, she would check the events or dealings by calling the phone numbers she obtained through Google, and they almost always checked out. There were

---

11 Michelle has mentioned her full name as a warning to anyone else who might fall into her trap.

a couple of things that didn't stack up, but perhaps because she really didn't want to believe she was wrong, she didn't pay them any heed. Gradually, her bank account was drained. She took out loans, borrowed on her credit cards and even took £5000 out of her business account.

Then one day, bingo! It finally hit home that she was indeed the victim of a very sophisticated scam. Something Suzanna said suddenly didn't sound right, and when Michelle checked up on it, it didn't tally. "Why it didn't dawn on me before, I will never know," sighed Michelle. Aren't we all guilty, though, of refusing to see what is right in front of us when we really don't want to acknowledge that someone we thought or hoped we could trust abuses us?

From the beginning, ZW was aware that Michelle had given Suzanna money, so she unceremoniously dumped her. Though their parting was acrimonious, in the end Michelle was relieved, as it was another weight around her neck that she could let go of.

After finally accepting that she had been scammed, Michelle contacted the police again. Though they were sympathetic, they were not surprised at what had happened. When they asked how much she had lost, the realisation that she now had no money hit Michelle hard. Altogether she had lost a massive £158,250. She became suicidal. The police issued an Extreme Risk Protection Order for Michelle, alerting the emergency services that she was a high suicide risk.

As the end of April 2019 drew near, Michelle began to optimistically anticipate the arrival of a VAT refund for her business. She called the VAT office to ask when she would receive the payment, only to be told that she had missed the deadline for the first quarter and would have to wait another three months to get the refund. This news was too much for Michelle to handle and her optimism plummeted towards the pessimistic apex. She told the person she was talking to, quite flippantly, that she might as well kill herself. In shock, the tax officer she was talking to asked her to repeat what she'd just said, which she did, then thinking nothing more about it drove into Wellingborough.

As she was leaving Earls Barton, Michelle noticed a police car with lights and sirens blaring travelling at high speed into the village. Even though that wasn't an everyday sight in the quiet village, she thought no more of it. Three minutes later her phone rang. It was the police. Standing outside her house, they wanted to know where she was. Her flippant remarks to the VAT office had generated a 999 call to the police with her address and contact details. The police officer insisted that she return home, and after a little argument, she gave in and returned. After escorting Michelle into the house, they were keen to know what was going on. Michelle explained about the scam that had led to her money troubles and hence the call to the VAT office. Even though she gave them the name of the detective she had reported the scam to and all the relevant information, the officers insisted on taking Michelle to Northampton General Hospital for assessment.

Arriving at the hospital with two police officers in tow didn't look good, but Michelle was beyond caring. After they had checked her in and departed, Michelle was then told that the mental health team wouldn't see her, so she ended up getting a taxi home barely 30 minutes after arriving under escort!

Chapter 29

With Friends Like These...

AFTER SHE RETURNED HOME, Michelle began to accept and understand the gravity of her situation. She had lost over £158,000! She had £400 left in her private bank account, but her business account was overdrawn to its limit. She had bills to pay but no way of paying them. She was, she thought, well and truly stuffed! Having some control over her thoughts, she turned not to suicide, but help, and went to a 'female only' crisis café in Northampton, where she explained her predicament to the nurse on duty. Though she was sympathetic and did her best to assure her that things would work out in the end, Michelle just couldn't see it. Her immediate solution was to give Michelle two coupons for a food bank on the outskirts of Northampton. Michelle couldn't believe she was actually going to get a food parcel.

The following day—a Friday—Michelle found the food bank located inside a church. She was given a free coffee and a slice of toast whilst she told them the kind of foods she liked. The caring volunteers set about making up two carrier bags full of her type of food—enough to last her for three days.

Even though they were no longer together, 31 years of marriage meant that Sue and Michelle still cared about one another. Michelle explained her dire situation to her ex, who very kindly lent her £2,000 to help her get her life back together. Michelle also phoned her brother, who lives in Spain, and after some heated discussions, he lent her business £500.

Before she was scammed, Michelle had taken out equity release on her house, but that sum of money was now lost. She contacted the broker who had sorted the equity release and asked if she could borrow some more. When he asked why, Michelle told him. It caused another problem. The broker's firm contacted their regulatory body and were advised that in their opinion Michelle lacked capacity to make decisions around her finances. To obtain further funds, which was possible, she would have to get her brother to make the decisions for her. One might see how a financial institution would be wary, but for Michelle, all it did was slow down the process of getting the additional £50,000 she needed to pay off some of the debts she had accrued.

After some weeks the further £50,000 was released on equity and Michelle was able to pay off the loans and overdrafts she had run up. She still had about £13,000 on a credit card, so she spread that between two other cards, paying a few hundred off each one every month. Even now, February 2021, Michelle still has some £6000 of credit card debt, but it is going down month by month. She does have enough money saved up now, so could pay the cards off if she wanted to, but as they are on a zero-interest balance transfer scheme, there is no need to pay them off totally just yet. Besides, paying them off might have a detrimental effect on her credit score, whereas making regular interest-free payments would not.

Michelle continued working, so still had an income. She gradually rebuilt her life and finances and got back into a comfortable situation. To increase her monthly income, she also took on a second lodger to join her first lodger—friend and former employee, SA—and herself in sharing the house.

Around about the time the scam started, Michelle had been accepted into a local LGBT (lesbian, gay, bisexual and transgender) social group. Members who knew Michelle well were sympathetic to her problems, and she was invited to join their steering committee to help set up the Wellingborough Pride event for August 2019. It was good for Michelle, as it gave her something positive to focus on, got her out of the house and in amongst friends. Or so she thought.

The Pride event, Michelle thought, was well organised, but being held in an old persons' day-care centre about a mile from the town centre, it was not the best location. If people didn't have their own transport, it was also not very accessible. Nevertheless, the sun shone and around three hundred people attended. It was a fortuitous day and the beginning of a new partnership for Michelle, as it was here that she met SR and his partner JM, who were promoting SR's book about his transition from female to male. Michelle struck up a conversation with them, and they all got along fine.

At the end of the day, the LGBT group set to dismantling everything and putting the chairs and tables away, and Michelle's two new friends departed. In the evening, the group celebrated their successful day with a buffet and disco. "It was good to unwind and have some 'us' time," Michelle recalls.

She didn't see SR again until late September/early October, when he attended a gender clinic development team meeting that Michelle was part of. During the meeting they both concluded that they could offer a service that the gender clinic had mentioned, but for which they had neither the resources nor the staff.

Michelle and SR agreed to meet at a pub to discuss their thoughts in more detail, and it wasn't long before they decided to set up in business together. SR had a Facebook support group by the name of 'Trans'pirational', and it was agreed that their company name would be 'Trans'pirational Ltd'. Whilst he set up the company with Companies House, Michelle got business cards printed in preparation for their new support services to trans people going live.

With little or no start-up budget, Michelle decided to use Facebook to advertise their business, utilising as many trans groups as she could find, as well as some LGBT groups, all over England. Soon the pair were receiving requests to hold support workshops at various locations and it looked as though they were going to be successful. Then Michelle got trolled!

A trans person in Leicester didn't like SR and took issue with the way Michelle was promoting the business. He started getting personal, and with her self-esteem on a knife edge, she, like a fool, retaliated. It just made matters worse. Then the troll turned his aggression on Michelle directly and two other trans people joined in. Michelle was fighting a losing battle. She was also getting drawn further and further into verbal suicide. In the end she broke off communications, but it was too late. The trolls copied and pasted some of Michelle's retaliatory comments into other sites, drumming up hatred towards both 'Trans'pirational' and her.

SR had been at work whilst this abusive social media outburst was going on, and when Michelle talked to him about it later, he was not best pleased. Michelle doesn't quite know what he did, but the whole matter got sorted. Nevertheless, she was left badly hurt. SR, his partner and a friend of theirs went round to Michelle's house that evening to see if she was okay and to talk her down. Though she seemed okay on the outside, she was in a terrible state on the inside. Their friend had connections to mental health services, and he gave Michelle his contact number in case she ever needed to talk.

With Michelle seemingly all right, the three left close to midnight. Left alone, Michelle began ruminating on what had happened and remonstrated with herself for being so stupid as to get embroiled in an online argument. Events weighed heavily on her and triggered feelings of suicide. By now, deep in a depression, she made the decision to end her life, as she had badly let her friends down. She overdosed. This time she didn't call 999 for help immediately after because she didn't want to be saved. Instead, and perhaps because a subliminal part of her brain thought otherwise, she sent a text to the friend of SR who had given her his number. She thought that he would be asleep and wouldn't get the text until the next morning, when it would be too late. She was wrong. He was still up. He called her immediately, asking what she had done. Then either he or Michelle, she cannot recollect, called 999. Michelle vaguely remembers the ambulance arriving, but her next memory was being at home two days later.

On that first night at home her friends, SR and JM, turned up with two others from the LGBT group. Michelle was still not 100 per cent in this world, as one of the tablets she had overdosed on were tranquilisers, and she was still feeling the after effects.

The two people from the LGBT group told Michelle not to go to any of their social events for two or three months, but being not quite with it, she didn't properly understand their meaning. A couple of days later, Michelle called them and asked what they had said and why they had said it. She was told again not to attend any socials for three months and was publicly removed from the steering committee. No reasons were given. The silence more than the act really upset Michelle. She requested the return of some things of hers and asked again why she was being treated like a criminal when she hadn't done anything to them or the group. Vulnerable and confused, she kept asking for answers and got nowhere. She was then reported to the police for harassment! The two representatives of the group then emailed Michelle to inform her that any further communication had to go via the group email address. She emailed as requested, and was once again reported to the police for harassment. Michelle felt hurt and confused. She was only doing as they asked and was only trying to make sense of what they were thinking and feeling. After all, how could she fix things if she didn't know what exactly had been broken? Effectively, she supposed, she had been kicked out of the LGBT group for something that did not, as far as she could see, affect them.

Feeling powerless, Michelle sought legal advice for discrimination and victimisation. After several months, the group paid out a lump sum so that she wouldn't take things further. Though she 'won', it was a hollow victory for Michelle.

Whilst this was going on, in November 2019 her old 'friend', ZW, got in touch by text to see if they could be friends again. Michelle was unsure, as things had ended badly previously, but agreed to meet her at a coffee shop in Northampton. Going with the intention of only staying for half an hour or so, ZW was very friendly and things went well, so they chatted for about three hours. ZW didn't want a relationship but wanted Michelle's friendship. Seeing no harm in this, Michelle started going out perhaps once a week for a coffee or to an antique centre with her. She told her what had happened on Facebook and with the LGBT group, and ZW found it hard to accept. Nonetheless, their friendship continued and things returned to almost where they were before. Once again, ZW sometimes stayed over in the spare room at Michelle's house and all was fine.

Then in March 2020 the first Covid-19 lockdown happened. ZW had had an operation on her foot and couldn't get out on her crutches on her own, so Michelle did her shopping for her each week. Things continued on an even keel until on 13 June Michelle was taken to hospital with terrible pains on the left side of her ribs. Fearing the worst, as it was really painful, she had a scan. It wasn't a heart attack, but the scan revealed a lump on Michelle's spine. With a diameter of about two to two and a half centimetres, Michelle was told it was a tumour, which was pressing on her spinal nerves, causing the pain she was experiencing.

Immediately, her thoughts turned to cancer. She wasn't scared and frightened, as she had put herself into very dangerous situations with each overdose she'd taken, but she was concerned. In need of a friend, she called ZW, but on getting no answer, sent her a text. She received no reply. Thinking that ZW must be asleep, she didn't try to contact her until the next day, Sunday 14 June, when she sent her a WhatsApp message. ZW blocked her. Now Michelle knew something was wrong, but not what. To try to get to the bottom of it, she sent her an email from an address she didn't often use. Still nothing.

WITH FRIENDS LIKE THESE . . .

The following Monday was Michelle's 65th birthday. She received a call from the police saying that ZW had reported her for harassment and that she wasn't to contact her ever again. Michelle was dumbstruck. ZW knew Michelle had a tumour, as she'd mentioned it in her first text, but in spite of that, she chose to dump Michelle on her birthday—she assumes, because of it. Of course, it's impossible to know what goes through another person's mind, and when someone you have been close to suddenly stops communicating, it can be very hard to come to terms with why they would behave like that. ZW had her own mental health issues and possibly couldn't cope with the idea that Michelle might have a serious physical illness which would have affected their relationship. Michelle had confided in her, and so she knew about the previous reports the LGBT group had made against her friend. Perhaps her way of dealing with the enormity of what might be wrong with Michelle meant that she couldn't invest any further in their relationship. Perhaps knowing that such a report would make Michelle look bad was a way of soothing her own complicated feelings. And so, Michelle's friendship was over again, but this time for good. Michelle couldn't countenance renewing things with her again after the way ZW had ended it. Michelle's tumour was further investigated and an MRI scan proved it was, after all, a harmless cyst.

In December 2019 Michelle had let it be known that she and SR were willing to give a talk on their personal transition journeys to members of the mental health teams based at Kettering and Northampton General Hospitals. Her suggestion was eagerly taken up, and in January the pair delivered a ninety-minute talk to both teams at a conference room in Berrywood Hospital. It went really well and they were asked to deliver a talk to the CRISIS team and other mental health workers at the mental health clinic meeting room in Corby. They delivered this on 7 February and 17 February 2020. It was so well received that they even received a standing ovation at one session.

During the first COVID-19 lockdown, they were unable to offer any further face-to-face talks, but it got Michelle thinking. If these three groups had liked what they were delivering, why didn't they do it properly? So in August 2020, National Gender Training was set up.

National Gender Training Logo

In December 2020, in speaking with the London Transgender Clinic, Michelle was told to stop taking oestrogen tablets and to use oestrogel. The reason being? The tablets cause blood clots. It hadn't occurred to Michelle before then, but now it all fitted into place. She'd taken her first three-month trial of oestrogen tablets in the first part of 1993 and had her first blood clots in the same period. She started taking the tablets during 2006/2007, and the blood clots had been ongoing since then.

When Michelle contacted her local gender clinic and explained what she had been told, the doctor readily agreed and confirmed that tablets have a much higher risk of blood clots. She also found out recently (February 2021) that the haematology department at Kettering General Hospital had told the same thing to the gender clinic on many occasions, but nothing was done. It begs the question: Why?

Oestrogel does carry the same risk, but it's a very small risk. Are the gender clinic and the NHS at fault? That is a question for another day.

Chapter 30

This is Me . . . In a Good Place

ANYONE WHO REALLY KNOWS Michelle can tell immediately that she has a heart of gold. She is empathic, intelligent, capable and someone who has the vision to see how society can benefit from small changes so that all individuals are able to live their best lives. Though she has undoubtedly been vulnerable throughout her life, she is amazingly resilient. She has throughout her 65 years on this planet, like the rest of us, made some mistakes, and perhaps even some grave errors of judgement. Not knowing who you really are is bound to have that effect. During her stays in different mental health hospitals, the staff

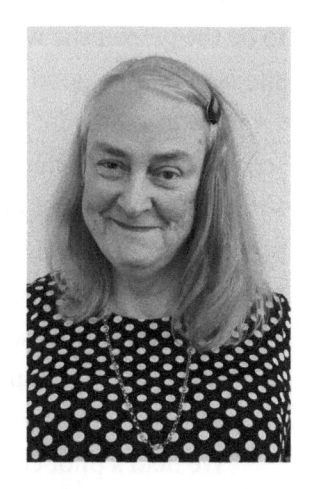

Me now March 2021

often said to her that she should write a book about her life. Perhaps it was said off the cuff or because they thought it might be cathartic, or perhaps because they could see that by writing about her life, she would in some small way be able to help others who are transitioning, or those around them, to understand just how difficult it can be.

Michelle decided to write this book in the third person. It is an autobiography because the events described herein are her lived experience: the words based on what she told or wrote and which were fashioned into the book by HK. Writing from the perspective of a third person played one other role: that of Michelle asking who she is. Quite often it felt like she was on the outside looking in—as a narrator might do—at other times she was well and truly aware of who she was, whether that was Michael or Michelle. It has taken a long time chronologically and emotionally for Michelle to be the person she wants and needs to be. But now, in May 2021, she is here, in a good place.

"I wanted to develop a course that was more than our life stories. It had to include everything about being trans. I researched some things, but most of it I knew already. I developed a PowerPoint presentation of some fifty-plus slides, including language and terminology, intersex, non-binary, pronouns, equality in the workplace and important legislation. SR gave me the information needed to cover his transition and the important stages within that pathway, and I did the same for the male-to-female route.

"We held a pilot course with some volunteers from the NHFT Recovery College and it was a huge success. I had reckoned on it being three hours, but it actually took three and a half. Next up was to get the course recognised as a Continuing Professional Development course (CPD). I used the London-based CPD

Accreditation services, and we achieved full accreditation at the beginning of September 2020.

"Now the hard work started: canvassing businesses and organisations to try to generate interest and income. I spent a lot of time emailing and talking to the ambulance services, police and fire services, the local NHS (NHFT) and some local businesses, and interest grew.

"I set our first full presentation for 14 December 2020, and we had representation from all the emergency services, as well as the Nautical Institute. The day soon arrived, and SR and I were a bit nervous but raring to go.

"Well! It was a huge success with everyone. We had fantastic feedback and picked up ongoing work for when the lockdown was lifted.

"Since then we have been running courses once a month, all with the same responses. We had meetings with different organisations that had attended, and plans were made for running training sessions once the pandemic situation allowed it.

"As a member of the Nautical Institute (NI), I proposed to write three articles for inclusion in their *Seaways* magazine, which they agreed to publish. The first article was in the February 2021 issue, with the next two in the following two months. Not wanting to stop there, I have now written articles for other magazines and am slowly introducing the awareness of being transgender to the wider public.

"I have also applied for Nautical Institute accreditation, as it is hoped that the three articles will generate international interest, and having NI accreditation would be crucial.

"Going forward, I am now training two other trans people up to run training courses on my behalf; plus, I am developing other courses dealing with bullying and harassment in the workplace, and blindness awareness. Marine Chart Services continues to thrive, selling vintage and antique nautical charts, and I am taking a friend on, part time, to help run the business for when the gender training starts.

"In my personal life, I'm now one month into a stable relationship. I'm more content now, much less focused on destructive thoughts and keen to progress my new career in transgender equality. In short, I have found happiness again."

Klinefelter Syndrome

KLINEFELTER SYNDROME (KS) is a condition that occurs in males when they have an extra X chromosome. Some males with KS have no obvious signs or symptoms, while others may have varying degrees of cognitive, social, behavioural and learning difficulties. Adults with KS may also have primary hypogonadism (decreased testosterone production), small and/or undescendent testes (cryptorchidism), enlarged breast tissue (gynecomastia), tall stature and/or inability to have biological children (infertility), as well as an abnormal opening of the penis (hypospadias) and a small penis (micropenis). KS is not inherited, but usually occurs as a random event during the formation of reproductive cells (eggs and sperm) that results in the presence of one extra copy of the X chromosome in each cell (47, XXY). KS treatment is based on the signs and symptoms present in each person. Life expectancy is usually normal, and many people with KS have a normal life. There is a very small risk of developing breast cancer and other conditions, such as a chronic inflammatory disease, called systemic lupus erythematosus.

The signs and symptoms of KS vary among affected people. Some men with KS have no symptoms of the condition or are only mildly affected. In these cases, they may not even know that they are affected by KS. When present, symptoms may include:

- small, firm testicles
- delayed or incomplete puberty, with lack of secondary sexual characteristics, resulting in sparse facial, body or sexual hair, a high-pitched voice and body fat distribution resulting in a rounder lower half of the body, with more fat deposited in the hips, buttocks and thigh instead of around the chest and abdomen
- breast growth (gynecomastia)
- reduced facial and body hair
- infertility
- tall stature
- abnormal body proportions (long legs, short trunk, shoulders equal to hip size)
- learning disability
- speech delay
- cryptorchidism
- opening (meatus) of the urethra (the tube that carries urine and sperm through the penis to the outside) on the underside of the penis (hypospadias) instead of the tip of the head of the penis
- social, psychological and behavioral problems

Source: GARD

Emotionally Unstable Personality Disorder

BORDERLINE PERSONALITY DISORDER (BPD), also known as emotionally unstable personality disorder (EUPD), is a mental illness characterised by a long-term pattern of unstable relationships, distorted sense of self and strong emotional reactions. Those affected often engage in self-harm and other dangerous behavior.

Causes: Unclear
Complications: Suicide
Treatment: Behavioural therapy

BPD is characterised by the following signs and symptoms:

- markedly disturbed sense of identity
- frantic efforts to avoid real or imagined abandonment, and extreme reactions to such
- splitting (black-and-white thinking)

Source: Wikipedia

In layman's terms, EUPD/BPD causes rapid mood swings, with often dangerous or suicidal impulses. The smallest of things can trigger it. Someone with this condition is generally vulnerable and can easily be coerced into foolish behaviour.

Acknowledgements and Thanks

Sir William Reardon Smith & Sons Ltd
Northamptonshire Healthcare Foundation Trust
MIND Northampton
MIND Kettering
NHFT Planned Care and Recovery Team (North)
NHFT UCAT
East Midlands Ambulance Service Trust
Northampton General Hospital
Kettering General Hospital
NHFT Gender Identity Clinic
Sue Clarke—my wife for 31 years

Contact Information

National Gender Training: www.nationalgendertraining.co.uk
Marine Chart Services: www.chartsales.co.uk
Helen Kelly Independent Celebrant Life Storywriter:
    www.helenkellycelebrant.co.uk